HORMONE REPLACEMENT THERAPY AND QUALITY OF LIFE

HORMONE REPLACEMENT THERAPY AND QUALITY OF LIFE

Edited by

Hermann P.G. Schneider MD, PhD, FRAM

Professor of Obstetrics and Gynecology
University of Muenster
Germany

The Parthenon Publishing Group
International Publishers in Medicine, Science & Technology

A CRC PRESS COMPANY
BOCA RATON   LONDON   NEW YORK   WASHINGTON, D.C.

Library of Congress Cataloging-in-Publication Data
Data available on request

Published in the USA by
The Parthenon Publishing Group
345 Park Avenue South
10th Floor
New York, NY 10010, USA

Published in the UK and Europe by
The Parthenon Publishing Group
23–25 Blades Court, Deodar Road
London SW15 2NU, UK

British Library Cataloguing in Publication Data
Data available on request

ISBN 1842140140

Typeset by H & H Graphics, Blackburn, UK

Printed and bound by
Bookcraft (Bath) Ltd., Midsomer Norton, UK

Contents

List of contributors

Elizabeth M. Alder PhD C Psychol FBPsS
Faculty of Health & Life Sciences
Napier University
74 Canaan Lane
Edinburgh EH9 2TB
UK

Hermann M. Behre MD
Department of Urology
Division of Andrology
University of Halle
Magdeburger Straße 16
06097 Halle/Saale
Germany

Aila Collins PhD
Department of Clinical Neuroscience
Karolinska Hospital
171 76 Stockholm
Sweden

**Lorraine Dennerstein AO MBBS PhD
   FRANZCP DPM**
Office for Gender and Health
Department of Psychiatry
Royal Melbourne Hospital
Charles Connibere Building
Parkville, Vic. 3050
Australia

Nancy Fugate Woods PhD RN FAAN
University of Washington School of Nursing
Box 357260
University of Washington
Seattle
WA 98195-7260
USA

J. G. Greene PhD
Department of Psychological Medicine
University of Glasgow
Academic Centre, Gartnavel Royal Hospital
1055 Great Western Road
Glasgow G12 0XH
UK

Janet Guthrie BSc MSc Dip Ed PhD
Office for Gender and Health
Department of Psychiatry
Royal Melbourne Hospital
Charles Connibere Building
Parkville, Vic. 3050
Australia

Lothar A. J. Heinemann MD DSc
ZEG-Centre for Epidemiology and Health
Research Berlin
Invalidenstrasse 115
10115 Berlin
Germany

Myra S. Hunter PhD C Psychol
Department of Psychology
Adamson Centre for Mental Health
Guy's, Kings & St Thomas' Medical Schools
St Thomas' Hospital
Lambeth Palace Road
London SE1 7EH
UK

Britt-Marie Landgren
Department of Obstetrics and Gynecology
Huddinge University Hospital
Karolinska Institute
Stockholm
Sweden

Anne M. Mariella RN MPH PhD
School of Nursing
Pacific Lutheran University
Tacoma WA 98447-0003
and
Co-Investigator, Seattle Midlife Women's
   Health Study
Box 357262
University of Washington
Seattle
WA 98195-7262
USA

Pasi Pöllänen MD PhD
Department of Obstetrics and Gynecology
University of Turku
20520 Turku
Finland

Farid Saad MD
Department of Clinical Research and
    Development
Jenapharm GmbH & Co KG
Otto-Schott-Straße 15
07745 Jena
Germany

Hermann P. G. Schneider MD PhD FRAM
Department of Obstetrics and Gynecology
University of Muenster
Von-Esmarch-Straße 56
ZMBE
48149 Muenster
Germany

York F. Zöllner PharmD MSc (Health Econ)
Department of Social Pharmacy
Pharmaceutical Institute
Humboldt University Berlin
Goethe Straße 54
13086 Berlin
Germany

Preface

Health and health-related quality of life (QoL) are no longer seen as being related only to physical health and absence of illness. In 1993, the World Health Organization defined QoL as "individuals' perceptions of their position of life in the context of the culture and value systems in which they live and in relation to their goals, standards and concerns." (WHO Division of Mental Health. *WHO-QOL study protocol: the development of the World Health Organization quality of life assessment instrument (MNG/PSF/93)*. Geneva: World Health Organization, 1993.) This definition is very broad and includes domains such as physical health, psychological state, level of independence, social relationships, environmental features and spiritual concerns. In the context of the menopause and changes that might occur as a result of hormone replacement therapy (HRT), we might expect alteration particularly in the domains of physical and psychological health as well as social relationships. Measuring the symptom dimension of QoL would imply an assessment of a subjective expression or manifestation of the underlying physical, psychological or social dysfunction. These are, in fact, evidence of *dis*-ease. Many women – during the menopause transition – are experiencing such dysfunction.

There have been multiple attempts at measuring QoL in order to provide objective assessment of a person's functioning. More recent questionnaires included measures of the individual's perceived health status or well-being. Life satisfaction, feelings of well-being, and the achievement of individual goals and expectations may be seen as a positive measure of QoL, while symptom severity and level of impairment by handicaps may reflect its loss. Attempts to objectify the variation of QoL will draw on knowledge of psychology, statistics, culture and clinical issues.

Highly experienced and internationally well-reputed experts present their views on the phase of life that encompasses the transition from the reproductive stage to a period of aging marked by waning gonadal function. The methodological aspects of assessing QoL, a review of the existing general and menopause-specific scales to measure the symptom dimension of QoL, and the most recent instruments for its contemporary evaluation specific for both women and men, are presented. Particular focus is given to depressed mood, sexuality and psycho-social factors with their association to the use of HRT. Importantly, a special chapter tackles health economics and evaluates the cost-effectiveness and cost-utility of HRT.

In recent years, there has been a growing awareness among clinicians of the importance of learning how patients cope with climacteric transition. Direct questioning is a simple and appropriate way of accruing information about how patients feel and function. Using standardized questionnaires ensures well-documented psychometric properties. For routine application and clinical practice or in clinical trials, it is essential that the instruments employed are simple and comparatively short. The majority of patients or probands welcome the opportunity to report how symptoms and subsequent treatment affect daily life. Psychometrically evaluated questionnaires allow uniform administration and unbiased quantification of data, as the response options are predetermined and thus equal for all respondents. A core set of questionnaires will allow the comparison of study results in patient populations.

The growing interest in the subjective aspects of QoL outcomes is evident from the increasing number of publications in this area. A growing emphasis has been on self-administered questionnaires. Unless conventional variables are supplemented with self-assessment measures, a limited picture of the impact of treatment on symptoms is obtained. The application of health-related QoL instruments requires the same scrutiny and application as the measurement of physiological outcomes. Random and representative samples of the population should be investigated in sufficient numbers and over prolonged periods of time. In terms of statistics, QoL is, by definition, a multi-state attribute. The use of many measures in the multiple statistical tests reduces the statistical power of the analysis. Health-related QoL certainly is a multi-dimensional concept, and there is a continuing debate on whether or not the aggregation of several dimensions into a summary index is appropriate. A summary score may falsely suggest improvement in one vital area and conceal deterioration in another. Indices, however, are practical, and are a convenient method of information transfer.

The editor and invited authors have covered the subject of QoL and its relationship to HRT to the extent that the readership is expected to gain a thorough, generalized grounding in an important health issue of growing global interest.

I am most grateful to all of the authors who contributed their chapters in due time such that Parthenon could have this book launched on the occasion of the 10th Anniversary of the International Menopause Society's triennial World Congress 2002 in Berlin. My special gratitude is with David Bloomer, Jean Wright and Stephen Nicholls not only for having suggested the project but also for their continuing editorial support, superb lectorate and excellent print.

Hermann P. G. Schneider

How to assess quality of life: problems and methodology

1

E. M. Alder

INTRODUCTION

There are many ways of assessing quality of life (QoL), something many health professionals may need to do. For example, clinicians may find such assessments useful[1] and health economists use the quality-adjusted life year (QALY) to plan healthcare provision[2]. Not all definitions of QoL are appropriate to the use in trials of hormone replacement therapy (HRT). HRT is most often used during the menopausal transition when menopausal symptoms become troublesome, although there is an increasing emphasis on its long-term use as prophylaxis. The effects on QoL may be important in attempts to maintain adherence with long-term use.

Some approaches to measuring QoL have been developed for disease-specific conditions and others are generic; only some of these may be appropriate to studies of HRT and the menopause. QoL can be seen positively in terms of life satisfaction and feelings of well-being, and goals and expectations that have been achieved. It may also be seen as reflecting symptom severity, level of impairment or handicap, or reflecting loss. QoL can be described in terms of subjective well-being (does your health interfere with your social life?) or functional status (can you dress unaided?).

Assessing QoL draws on knowledge of psychology, statistics, culture and clinical issues. Health psychology has tried to address issues of health outcomes of therapy in the broadest sense and the effectiveness of any therapy cannot be measured in physical terms alone[3]. Therefore QoL in the menopause can be measured in terms of symptoms, personal experience or functional ability. In attempting to measure QoL in the menopause and, in particular, in studies of HRT, several problems require consideration.

QUALITY OF LIFE IN GENERAL

There is no universally accepted definition of quality of life; every study seems to use a different one and, as we can see from this volume, it is a very broad concept. Bowling[4] discusses some of the issues.

Health status and QoL are not linearly related, and measurement of health is not a proxy for measuring QoL. Health-related QoL may refer to the effects of an individual's physical state on their psychosocial functioning, but this may be too limited. Hunt and McKenna[5] pointed out that there was no agreed definition, no theoretical base, inappropriate use of measures, lack of recognition of the social basis of definitions and measurement and confusion with QoL and quality of care.

In 1946 the World Health Organization (WHO)[6] defined health as "complete physical, mental and emotional well-being". Health-related QoL is no longer seen as being about only physical health and an absence of illness. In 1993, the WHO defined QoL[7] as "individuals' perceptions of their position of life in the context of the culture and value systems in which they live and in relation to their goals, standards and concerns". The definition includes six domains: physical health, psychological state, levels of independence, social relationships, environmental features and spiritual concerns.

This approach is very wide, and in the context of the menopause and changes that might occur as a result of HRT, we might expect there to be different changes in different domains. Changes are particularly likely to be found in the domains of physical and psychological health and social relationships. The research that predates this definition tended to focus on symptomatology and symptomatic indices as measures of QoL. It would probably now be agreed that QoL is a multidimensional concept and includes both positive and negative aspects of life.

Early attempts at measuring QoL tried to provide an objective assessment of the person's functioning, whereas current questionnaires may include QoL measures of an individual's perceived health status or well-being. Assessing physical functioning might involve measuring the ability to perform specific tasks or the activities of daily living, and mental functioning in performing cognitive tasks and social interactions. These measures are probably not relevant to studies of HRT, where the level of physical and mental functioning is probably good to start with. The subjective appraisal of health may be more influenced by vasomotor symptoms experienced in the menopause and likely to be affected by HRT.

QoL can be also defined as "a reflection of the way that patients perceive and react to their health status and to other non-medical aspects of their lives"[8]. This aspect might be included in generic measures of QoL but not in lists of menopausal symptoms.

It is clear that the measurement of QoL is strongly influenced by its purpose[9]. Probably all health professions have a different approach (e.g. nurses, health economists, physicians), and their approach will be different again from the perspective of each patient. Ignoring these differences has led to methodological problems, some of which will be discussed below in relation to menopause and HRT.

Health professionals can objectively assess QoL, or it can be measured subjectively by individuals themselves. Some aspects of life are of universal importance but the weights attached to these will differ between and within cultures. Most scales are based on health professionals' ideas of what is relevant, and often on previous measures. Some domains will be specific to the individual, for example spiritual needs may be highly important to one person but not to another.

A paradox with measuring QoL is that patients who have significant health and functional problems do not necessarily have poor QoL scores. People with severe disabilities may report a good QoL despite having difficulties with activities of daily living and being socially isolated[10]. An individual approach has been taken in the Patient Generated Index of Quality of Life[11]. It asks people to generate their own list of five areas relating to QoL and allocate a value reflecting their relative importance. This allows individuals to generate their own priorities. So, for example, it would allow mobility to be considered more important than pain. It is probably particularly useful in assessing changes in areas of health that are more individually determined than societal. It may be less suitable for postal surveys but has intuitive appeal and may be very acceptable, thus increasing response rates.

Ratings of QoL made by individuals and their carers often do not correlate. The assessment of the QoL of menopausal women will be influenced by their past experience and their expectations for the future. Studies of HRT can take a long time, for example six or twelve months, which is a problem because QoL is not constant over time. People assess their health-related QoL by comparing their expectations with their experience[12]. If expectations match experience there is no impact on QoL but if experience (such as night sweats) is worse then there is an impact. Carr and colleagues[12] illustrate this with an example of back pain but it can be readily be translated into the onset of menopausal changes.

If a woman believes she should not have vasomotor symptoms, there is a gap between expectations and experience and she may be depressed. If she later accepts that vasomotor symptoms are part of the transition through the menopause, the discrepancy between expectations and experience is reduced and she will have a better QoL. If she is offered HRT, her expectation that she will be free from vasomotor symptoms will be raised, and, if the therapy is very effective, her experience will be greater than her expectations and we should expect a raised level of well-being. This illustrates that QoL is a dynamic construct and may change over the course of a clinical trial of HRT.

The three main methodological problems are: people have different expectations; they may be at different points on their menopausal transition; and the reference value of their expectations may change over time. The approach taken for assessing QoL depends on the question asked; if the question is whether HRT improves QoL, it must be further broken down into the relevant QoL domains. A simple outcome might be the reduction of vasomotor symptoms, and it might be expected this would enhance self-esteem and improve psychological health and social relations. However, if vasomotor symptoms were not a problem for the woman or if her psychological health was affected more by other factors, then HRT might not improve QoL, even if there was a significant reduction in symptoms. In large clinical trials, such individual differences may be hidden.

The contrast between the use of the medical model leading to an emphasis on symptom reduction, and a broader approach, has been very evident in measuring QoL in older people. The medical model leads to a search for a cure and the reduction or absence of symptoms, and thereby an increase in the level of functioning. This leads to a search for an objective measure of easily quantifiable functional criteria. In contrast to this traditional medical professional view, the older person may be more concerned with issues of self-identity, and preservation of meaning in life. Menopausal women are not ill and may not perceive themselves as unhealthy, yet they are moving into a transition that will lead inexorably to old age.

Brandstater and Greive[13] see the gradual aging process as leading to successive loss of control, and higher rates of depression (which may be associated with bereavement) and lower self-esteem (there is an emphasis on youth and beauty in Western society). They suggest that elderly people cope by moving through stages of assimilation, accommodation and using immunizing mechanisms. Although they developed this model to describe changes in QoL in elderly people, it is relevant to menopausal women. In assimilation, people maintain current activities, goals and aspirations. Menopausal women might make strong efforts to maintain fitness by taking exercise, preserve their attractiveness by using cosmetics and use aids such as reading glasses to achieve their goals. As the aging process continues, they replace current goals and aspirations with new ones. They give up difficult goals or reduce their level of expectations about their level of performance. Postmenopausal women may accept changes in hair colour and no longer expect to run marathons. Later they use immunizing mechanisms such as perceptual filtering where they attend to past achievements rather than their current state. It can be seen from this that QoL will change as a woman goes through the menopausal transition. There is no single state of normal health to which she can be restored. The effectiveness of HRT on her QoL may be greater when she first begins therapy than it might be later, which may be highly relevant to problems of maintaining adherence over long periods if HRT is prescribed for prophylaxis.

Improvement in health-related QoL may be the goal of the health professional, but some of the domains described by the WHO may be outside their control and area of expertise. It is arguable how concerned the health professional should be about the environmental features of QoL, although deprivation is important, and we know that inequalities of life are related to health. Similarly for the spiritual dimension, many health professionals feel that this is outside their remit or feel inadequately equipped to cope with people's spiritual needs. The dimensions that primarily concern them are physical health, psychological state and, to some extent, independence and social relationships. It is the first two that are often described as health status and these are usually the focus of attention in clinical trials of HRT. The physician who is trying to improve QoL for individual women may take into account these other dimensions, so the goal of therapy may amount to more than the alleviation of symptoms.

THE MENOPAUSAL TRANSITION

The whole process of transition from pre- to post-menopause may take over ten years. These ten years, which may begin any time from 40 to nearly 60 years of age, are also times of life changes and considerable psychological changes. There are changes in role. The woman may become less concerned with parenting her own children and perhaps more focused on her career; she may also have elderly parents that need care. Grandchildren may make more demands but also become a source of pleasure and satisfaction. There are social and psychological consequences of fractures in old age and consequent loss of mobility and independence, which directly affect QoL.

Menopause is not an illness, so the illness model is inappropriate for a psychosocial transition. Menopause may be regarded by women and society as an illness because age-related changes are expected, due to beliefs about illness and of attributions of symptoms.

People vary in their ability to report physiological states such as heart rate, and some will be more accurate in reporting hot flushes than others. And not all symptoms will necessarily be reported. Hot flushes may be perceived as part of a natural pattern of aging or as a symptom that requires medical attention, and the way in which these affect QoL may lead some women to consult physicians, but others to ignore them.

Changes that occur during the menopausal transition may be attributed to hormonal alterations and conceptualized as an illness (a hormone deficiency) requiring treatment. Illness is a psychological concept and has different meanings for different individuals. People often recognize that they are ill because of the presence of symptoms. If they experience unusual symptoms, which are severe enough and last for long enough, they may feel that they are ill and then behave in certain ways. This is called 'illness behavior'[14]. The awareness of symptoms depends on what else is going on around us and our expectations[15], and the perception of those symptoms depends on what we expect. If women have negative expectations of the menopause they are more likely to report negative experiences[16–18]. If hot flushes are perceived as a sign of aging, and as being very conspicuous to others, they will be more likely to be reported.

The effect of expectations on symptom reporting has been demonstrated experimentally[19]. Subjects in two different groups were told either that ultrasonic noise might cause an increase in skin temperature, or that it might cause a decrease. They were then told that they were listening to a tape of ultrasonic noise, although in fact it was blank. Actual skin temperature did not change, but fluctuations in temperature were reported as being cooler or warmer according to whether they had been told that skin temperature might decrease or increase. Mechanic[20] suggested that symptom reporting is influenced by the number and persistence of symptoms, the extent of the social and physical disability resulting from the symptoms, and the recognition and identification – and perceived severity of – the symptoms.

An example of the discrepancy between the perception of symptoms and medical reality is shown in the reporting of menstrual blood loss[21]. Reports of blood loss are unreliable when compared with objective measures of hemoglobin. If objective measures are taken and they do not agree with the reported loss, the patient may be dismissed as not having a gynecological problem. Although the hemoglobin content of blood in sanitary towels or tampons is a convenient and reliable measure of blood loss, it may not be the same as the volume of fluid loss. The woman may be more aware of the fluid loss and certainly more concerned about it. The amount of fluid that needs to be collected in tampons and towels is a salient symptom to the woman, but the loss of hemoglobin is salient to the gynecologist.

Similar reporting bias may occur in the reporting of vasomotor symptoms and they may be affected by skin type, clothing and ambient temperature. Vasomotor symptoms may or may not interfere with social activities. Hot flushes and night sweats in menopausal women may be perceived as normal, and not a medical problem, yet in some cases they cause severe social distress.

We are constantly seeking the meaning of events and changes in our bodies. These changes may be explicable in terms of the medical model, and have a clear physiological etiology and consequent treatment. But menopausal symptoms include many less-clearly defined psychological symptoms. These may be attributed to physical changes such as hot flushes, or may be seen as symptomatic of the menopause itself, and, by implication, a consequence of endocrinological changes. Symptoms on their own have no meaning and are merely bodily sensations. Different symptoms will be accounted for in different ways. A backache may be attributed to premenstrual syndrome, excessive gardening or old age depending on the individual's lifestyle. Symptoms are not static and their pattern may contribute to the search for meaning. Leventhal and Benyamini[22] suggest there is an asymmetrical relationship between the symptom and the diagnostic label. People with symptoms seek a diagnostic label. If they experience changes in mood or well-being, they may be reassured that they are experiencing the menopause. This is in spite of the lack of evidence of an association between mood and menopausal transition. People given a diagnosis may be more sensitive to symptoms if they are told that they are 'going through the menopause'. If they are aware that there is a syndrome called the menopause they may be alerted to symptoms.

We can only report a symptom if we have a name for it. The more we know, the more our awareness of potential symptoms, and changes in our health, increases. If someone is enrolled in a clinical trial of HRT they may only agree if they are experiencing severe symptoms. If they are asked to complete a symptom checklist, they may be alerted to possible menopausal symptoms of which they had not been previously aware. Symptom reporting may be related to a threshold or to a change. An increase in sleep disturbance or an increase in the aching of joints may be seen as a symptom and related to changes in menstrual patterns.

Individual assessments of QoL can help the health professional to become aware of the domains of life that can be affected by a health problem. Although a woman may consult because of reported vasomotor symptoms there may be an underlying depression. HRT may relieve the symptoms and relieve the depression, or there may be other factors affecting the depression which need further investigation. Sometimes the benefits of therapy on QoL can be indirect.

In a clinical trial of anti-hypertension therapy and management, a diet that resulted in weight loss had a greater effect on QoL than drug therapy, because weight reduction was more effective in reducing the physical symptoms than drug therapy and this was related to their satisfaction with life[23].

QUALITY OF LIFE ACROSS CULTURES

Culture can be defined in many ways: for example, a set of accepted ideas, practices, values and characteristics[24]. It defines a group of people that have a common identity. Most of us could identify our culture and it gives some structure to our lives. Cultural mores tell us how to behave in order to maintain and promote health and how to prevent illness or disease. The cultural beliefs that surround the menopause will influence people's views of health and are therefore determinants of QoL.

QoL can mean different things in different cultures, thus measurements of QoL cannot be used universally. Kagawa-Singer[25] found that Western measures were inadequate to detect cultural differences between Japanese-Americans and Anglo-Americans. Japanese-Americans saw the side-effects of cancer treatment to be expected and endured, whereas Anglo-Americans saw them as problems to be eliminated or overcome. Kagawa-Singer suggested that QoL universally includes the need for safety and security, a sense of integrity and a sense of belonging. These are concepts far removed from a list of menopausal symptoms. She found that disruption to the activities of daily living due to cancer was greater in Anglo men and Japanese women than in Japanese men and Anglo women, and this was related to their different expectations. In Nigeria it was found that most (60%) of women were glad to have reached the stage of menopause[26]. The most commonly reported serious problems were internal heat, abdominal/waist pain and weakness/fatigue. There were also marked differences within different ethnic groups. Similar emphasis on physical symptoms of aching backs rather than vasomotor symptoms were observed by the author in focus groups of menopausal women in Nepal and illustrate the problems of using measures across cultures.

Standardized measures of health-related QoL are almost necessarily laden with cultural values. Even if they are translated, back-translated and reviewed they may not be equivalent if they are based on invalid cross-cultural assumptions. Meadows[27] suggests that scales must have equivalence across cultures. The measures should have:

(1) content equivalence – the same information is covered for different cultural groups;

(2) semantic equivalence – different language versions should agree;

(3) technical equivalence – the procedure for administration, scaling, scoring, length and time to completion should be the same across groups;

(4) scalar equivalence – the measure is able to rank people from different language or cultural groups in equivalent ways; and

(5) criterion equivalence – the standard against which the measure is compared should be the same across groups.

The WHO Quality of Life Assessment (WHOQOL) used focus groups of health professionals, patients and people in the community in different countries to generate items. They were allocated into the six domains and analyzed nationally[28]. This enabled country-specific items to be added to the core items making a culture-specific measure.

Cultural and demographic differences have strong effects on health and its perceived relationship with QoL. Poor health may be an accepted part of living in some deprived areas, while affluence may bring increased expectations of health. More illness is found in community surveys in lower socio-economic groups, but people in higher socio-economic groups are more likely to seek health care. There are higher levels of morbidity in poorer countries but greater levels of health care in more affluent countries. Even within a culture, there are sub-cultural differences. Older people consult their doctors less often than younger people in relation to their level of illness[29].

With the life expectancy of women continuing to increase, women are spending more of their lives post menopause. This has led to suggestions that the use of HRT might increase in many countries, and to an interest in the QoL of older women. New measures of QoL-related domains have been developed, such as the Menopause Rating Scale (MRS) in Germany[30,31] and the Menopause-Specific QoL Questionnaire (MENQOL) in Canada[32]. In the United Arab Emirates, Bener and colleagues[33] used a translation of the MENQOL to assess menopause-specific QoL in a sample of 390 women aged 45–62, who were at least two years since their last period. The four domains of vasomotor, psychosocial, physical and sexual were confirmed but there were fewer menopausal symptoms than in Western countries, and fewer in women of lower education. The most frequently reported symptom was 'aches in back of neck or head' (46%) and only 33% reported hot flushes. However, many of these women would be well past the time of maximum endocrinologic change. In order to establish validity women would need to be assessed over the menopausal transition to detect changes.

PROBLEMS OF STANDARDIZED MEASURES

In clinical consultation there may be dislike of using questionnaires to measure something as elusive as QoL. Clinicians are used to receiving laboratory reports and to relying on their accuracy, although even hormone assays carry a margin of error. Not all scales are equally psychometrically sound and it is important to know the properties of reliability and validity of any scale that is used (see below). Scores on a scale only give an indication of the extent of a problem and are never a substitute for clinical judgement. The context may be very important and scales that include several of the dimensions described above are more likely to be useful than those which concentrate on only one.

A woman's reporting of symptoms to the clinician is dependent on her illness behavior and health beliefs. In collecting data in clinical trials of HRT, the data can be biased in many ways. Retrospective recall of data (for example, "How many hot flushes have you had in the last day/week/month?") can be influenced by the phrasing of the question – and the longer the period of recall, the greater the inaccuracy. Open-ended questions may elicit fewer symptoms than checklists. A symptom may be noticed (a sign) but not be either frequent or troublesome (a symptom worth reporting). In some epidemiological studies, the purpose is disguised as a general health survey so that stereotypes of the menopause are avoided. A widely used measure of menopausal symptoms is called the Women's Health Questionnaire (WHQ) although it focuses on menopausal health[18].

If QoL is assumed to be closely related to menopausal symptoms, the evidence for a relationship between menopausal status and QoL is conflicting. Some studies find that only vasomotor symptoms significantly increase over the menopausal transition[34] and are presumed to be hormone related. It follows that a measure of the physical domain of QoL (for example, of vasomotor symptoms) is more likely to show the effect of HRT than those that are more broadly based.

In a large cross-sectional study, over 4000 women aged 45–54 years were recruited through a women's magazine in the Netherlands in order to investigate the relationship between menopausal stage and menopausal symptoms[35]. The study found that only vasomotor symptoms and (to a lesser extent) loss of interest in sex were associated with menopausal status. QoL was measured by asking for the level of satisfaction with 17 life domains. These were factor-analyzed, giving four subscales of general life satisfaction, satisfaction with health and medical care, sexual satisfaction and satisfaction with social support. They were not related directly to menopausal status nor to vasomotor symptoms. Lower life-satisfaction and less satisfaction with social support were related to psychological symptoms measured on a Dutch translation of Greene's Climacteric Scale[36]. This minor increase in psychological morbidity associated with the transitional phase of the menopause rather than with the postmenopausal phase has been found in other studies[37]. But cross-sectional studies do not imply causation and we do not know which comes first.

The implied relationship of hormonal status to psychological symptoms is probably mediated by vasomotor symptoms and we have a 'domino effect'. Any reduction in vasomotor symptoms, whether occurring naturally over the transition to the postmenopausal phase or by intervention with HRT, is likely to have a beneficial effect on self-esteem and psychological well-being[38].

Menopause is a transition and differs from illness. Self identity may be determined by age-related changes, illness cognitions and symptom attributions. These need to be taken into account when assessing changes that affect QoL during the menopausal transition. Health status, measured by symptoms, and QoL are not linearly related and measurement of health is not a proxy for measuring QoL.

MEASUREMENT IN THE MENOPAUSE

Modern psychometrics has led to the publication of reliable and valid scales that can be used in research. A scale is based on a defined population and it is important to know whether it is a community or a clinic sample. Self reports are considered more valid and reliable than physician ratings. The language may influence reporting and there may be differences between British English and American English. A scale of menopausal symptoms should be based on factor analysis, which allows subscales to be produced. Scales used to measure symptoms or other domains of QoL must have certain psychometric properties, as described in standard psychological texts and more specialized textbooks[4,39,40].

Scales must have validity. They must measure what they are intended to measure (face validity) and must include factors that are clinically relevant (these should be self-evident). Content validity refers to whether the scale includes all relevant areas, and whether all items fall into one of these areas. Criterion validity reflects the correlation with a gold standard or superior measure. If there is no gold standard then an alternative is to ask whether the measure produces results that conform to a theory. A new scale is given together with one it is intended to replace. Of course, if there is near perfect agreement it is probably no improvement unless it is shorter, simpler or less expensive to administer. If it has criterion validity, it will also predict differences in the expected direction.

Most scales are based on theoretical constructs, and construct validity can be tested by assessing the extent to which the scale is related to other constructs and variables derived from the theory. This is usually established by factor analysis.

Modern scales need to show reliability, consistency and effectiveness. Does the measure produce the same results when repeated with the same subjects? Inter-rater (or inter-observer) reliability determines whether different observers obtain similar results, and test–retest reliability determines whether similar results are obtained at different points in time. The tests are given on two separate occasions and high correlations are expected. Internal reliability is usually measured by Cronbach's alpha; alphas below five suggest that the items are not tapping into the same area. For example, mood items should relate to each other but might be different from mobility. If there is high agreement between items, for example over nine, then it probably means that they are measuring the same thing.

Research studies on QoL are often carried out on patient populations or community samples, so the scale must be acceptable and simple to use. It must be short enough to be completed in a reasonable time. Questions must be in acceptable language and format and clearly laid out, and there must be no ambiguity in the scoring of responses. Font size and type of print can influence acceptability. The measure must be able to discriminate between different degrees of severity or detect changes that might occur following therapy. Patients who have progressive or advanced illness often score poorly on many QoL measures (known as a floor effect), because the measures rely heavily on assessing the patient's functioning as part of the assessment. In contrast, if symptoms are few and there is a high QoL there may be a ceiling effect so no improvement can be detected. The application of some of these principles to generic QoL scales is discussed by Muldoon and colleagues[41], and they conclude that conceptual and methodological issues have received insufficient attention and this constrains the interpretation of the current medical literature.

A good measure of menopausal symptoms would appear appropriate to menopausal women, would correlate positively with other scales, include relevant items such as libido and would distinguish between pre- and perimenopausal women. There would be a high correlation with scores on other measures of menopausal symptoms. There is no single right way to measure QoL; the measurement needs to be tailored to the aim of the assessment.

Hunt[42] suggests that studies of QoL in women give different results because there is no agreed definition of QoL, they use different measures, measures are not condition specific, populations differ and menopausal status is not consistently defined. If the physical domain of QoL is regarded as being the most important outcome of treatment by HRT, there are a number of symptoms measures which can be used to assess outcome. The Kupperman Menopausal Index was widely used in many early research studies in Europe and the USA[43]. The index combines self-report and physician ratings, but not measures of vaginal dryness and loss of libido, thus lacking content validity. The original publications gave no demographic data for the sample and weighting was used without statistical justification. The terms were ill-defined and many of them are archaic. The categories included overlapping scores, and most importantly scores were summed without being based on independent factors[44]. Since the original publications, many research studies have used modified versions, but they have not been validated.

Bowling[4] describes the concepts behind the measurement of QoL and gives detailed descriptions of several scales. QoL can be measured by asking the subject, their carer or their health professionals. The meaning of the measure will depend on who is the rater and the purpose of the measure. Assessments can be made by standardized questions, individualized questions and by standard scales. Standardized scales are most often used in research studies or in audit.

The WHOQOL has been developed internationally. It has six domains of 29 facets and has been used widely[45]. The Nottingham Health Profile[46] (NHP) is a simple scale and can be used in community studies, giving a very functional assessment. However, it is now more usual to have specific scales for specific conditions or social contexts. In menopause research, the Greene Climacteric Scale[36] and the WHQ[18] have been developed in the UK from clinic populations based on factor analysis, and have good psychometric properties. In Germany, the MRS[30] provides three subscales and makes good many deficiencies of the Kupperman index. It has good psychometric properties with high levels of reliability[31]. These scales are all symptom-based, but QoL research has taken a much broader view and is less illness-based.

There has been considerable research in the USA on the development of the SF36 scales with subsequent validation in the UK[47,48]. The SF36 provides eight subscales covering physical and social functioning, role limitations, pain, energy/vitality and general and mental health. It takes about ten minutes to complete and can be used in postal surveys. In a significant study[31] the SF36 was compared with other standardized scales in a study of over 300 women. It was found that the SF36 and MRS correlated negatively for both somatic and psychological symptoms. The more symptoms, the worse the QoL, but the correlations were strongest for psychological symptoms. The closest associations were found in the most and least severe menopausal symptoms, with the highest correlations in physical role functioning, bodily pain, vitality and emotional role functioning. However, all these items are interrelated and the scales were dominated by symptom reporting, reflecting the illness model. There was no attempt to individualize the menopausal experience and of course they are culturally dependent, reflecting Western concepts of health.

Menopausal status has been shown to be related to QoL using the NHP[49,50] and the WHQ[18]. However, other research has suggested that well-being in the menopause is more closely associated with psychosocial factors[51]. Jacobs and co-workers[52] developed a condition-specific questionnaire to assess QoL in menopausal women. They analyzed a 48-item questionnaire from over 1000 women aged 40–63, recruited from two English health authority lists and a national women's magazine. Items were derived from interviews and focus groups. Women reported their own menopausal status. Factor analysis revealed seven factors: sleep, energy, cognition, symptom impact, feelings, social interaction and appetite, which were combined to give a total menopausal quality of life score (MQOL).

Mean scores showed an inverted U-shaped pattern across the stages of the menopause, with lowest scores in the middle of the menopausal transition. The MQOL was highly correlated with a global QoL scale, QOL[53]. However, the subscales of social interaction and symptom impact showed a steady decline across the menopausal transition. If the end of the menopausal transition coincides with an increasing QoL, this may confound studies of the effect of HRT over time.

The problems and issues in measuring QoL in studies of the menopause and hormone replacement therapy are not unique, and measurement of quality of life is worth doing, if ultimately it has positive health outcomes for individual women.

References

1. Hopkins A. How might measures of quality of life be useful to me as a clinician? In Hopkins A, ed. *Measures of the Quality of Life and the Uses to Which Such Measures May be Put.* London: Royal College of Physicians, 1992
2. Williams A, Kind P. The present state of play about QALYs. In Hopkins A, ed. *Measures of the Quality of Life and the Uses to Which Such Measures May be Put.* London: Royal College of Physicians, 1992
3. Alder B. *Psychology of Health: Application of Psychology for Health Professionals*, 2nd edn. Amsterdam: Harwood Academic Publishers, 1999
4. Bowling A. *Measuring Health*, 2nd edn. Buckingham: Open University Press, 1997
5. Hunt S, McKenna S. Do we need measures other than QALYs? In Hopkins A, ed. *Measures of the Quality of Life and the Uses to Which Such Measures May be Put.* London: Royal College of Physicians, 1992
6. WHO. *Constitution of the WHO Geneva A.* Switzerland: World Health Organization, 1946
7. WHO Division of Mental Health. *WHO-QOL Study Protocol: the development of the World Health Organization quality of life assessment instrument (MNG/PSF/93).* Geneva: World Health Organization, 1993
8. Gill TM, Feinstein AR. A critical appraisal of the quality of quality-of-life measurements. *J Am Med Assoc* 1994;272:619–26
9. King CR, Hinds PS. *Quality of Life from Nursing and Patient Perspectives.* Sudbury: Jones and Bartlett Publishers, 1998
10. Albrecht GL, Devlieger PJ. The disability paradox: high quality of life against all odds. *Soc Sci Med* 1999;48:977–88
11. Ruta DA, Garratt AM, Leng M, *et al.* A new approach to the measurement of quality of life: the patient generated index (PGI). *Med Care* 1994;32:1109–26
12. Carr AJ, Gibson B, Robinson PG. Is quality of life determined by expectations or experience? *Br Med J* 2001;322:1240–3
13. Brandstater J, Greive W. The ageing self: stabilizing and protective processes. *Development Rev* 1994;14:52–80
14. Kasl SA, Cobb S. Health behavior, illness behavior, and sick role behavior. *Arch Environment Health* 1966;12:246–66
15. Pennebaker JW. *The Psychology of Physical Symptoms.* New York: Springer-Verlag, 1982
16. Avis NE, McKinlay SM. A longitudinal analysis of women's attitudes toward the menopause: results from the Massachusetts Women's Health Study. *Maturitas* 1991;13:65–79
17. Hunter M. The South-East England study of the climacteric and post menopause. *Maturitas* 1992;14:117–26
18. Hunter M. The Women's Health Questionnaire: a measure of mid aged women's perceptions of their emotional and physical health. *Psychol Health* 1992;7:45–54
19. Pennebaker JW, Skelton JA. Selective monitoring of physical sensations. *J Personality and Social Psychol* 1981;41:213–23
20. Mechanic D. *Medical Sociology*, 2nd edn. New York: Free Press, 1978
21. Granleese J. Personality, sexual behaviour and menstrual symptoms: their relevance to clinically presenting with menorrhagia. *Personality and Individual Differences* 1990;11:379–90
22. Leventhal H, Benyamini Y. Lay beliefs about health and illness. In Baum A, Newman S, Weinman J, *et al*, eds. *Cambridge Handbook of Psychology, Health and Medicine.* Cambridge: Cambridge University Press, 1997:72–7
23. Wassertheil-Smoller S, Blaufox MD, Oberman A, *et al.* Effect of hypertensives on sexual function and quality of life: the TAIM study. *Ann Intern Med* 1991;114:613–20
24. Stratton P, Hayes N. *A student's Dictionary of Psychology.* London: Edward Arnold, 1988
25. Kagawa-Singer M. Redefining health: living with cancer. *Soc Sci Med* 1993;37:295–304
26. Olawoye JE, Olarinde ES, Aderibigbe TO. *Women and Menopause in Nigeria.* Ibidan, Nigeria: SSRHN, 1998

27. Meadows K. Criteria for translations of health measurement instruments. *Quality Life Res* 1994;3:67

28. Skevington SM, Bradshaw J, Saxena S. Selecting national items for the WHOQOL: conceptual and psychometric consideration. *Soc Sci Med* 1999;48:473–87

29. Cartwright A. Medicine taking by people aged 65 or more. *Br Med Bull* 1990;46:63–76

30. Schneider HPG, Henineman LAJ, Rosemeier H-P, *et al.* The Menopause Rating scale (MRS): reliability of scores of menopausal complaints. *Climacteric* 2000;3:59–64

31. Schneider HPG, Henineman LAJ, Rosemeier H-P, *et al.* Menopause Rating scale (MRS): comparison with Kupperman index and quality-of-life scale SF-36. *Climacteric* 2000;3:50–8

32. Hilditch JR, Lewis J, Peter A, *et al.* A menopause-specific quality of life questionnaire: development and psychometric properties. *Maturitas* 1996;24:161–75

33. Bener A, Rizk DE, Shaheen H, *et al.* Measurement specific quality of life satisfaction during the menopause in an Arabian Gulf country. *Climacteric* 2000;3:43–9

34. WHO. *Research on the Menopause in the 1990s (Technical Research series)*. Geneva: World Health Organization, 1996

35. Vanwesenbeeck I, Vennix P, van de Wiel H. 'Menopausal symptoms': associations with menopausal status and psychosocial factors. *J Psychosom Obstet Gynecol* 2001;22:149–58

36. Greene JG. *Guide to the Greene Climacteric Scale.* Glasgow: University of Glasgow, 1991

37. Hunter MS. Emotional wellbeing, sexual behaviour and hormone replacement therapy. *Maturitas* 1990;12:299–314

38. Alder EM, Ross LA, Gebbie AE. Menopausal symptoms and the domino effect. *J Reprod Infant Psychol* 2000;18:75–8

39. Jenkinson C, McGee H. *Health Status Measurement.* Oxford: Radcliffe Medical Press, 1998

40. Rust J. Golombok S. *Modern Psychometrics. The Science of Psychological Assessment.* London: Routledge, 1989

41. Muldoon MF, Barger S, Flory JD, *et al.* What are quality of life measurements measuring? Br Med J 1998;316:542–5

42. Hunt SM. The problem of quality of life. *Quality Life Res* 1997;6:205–12

43. Blatt MH, Weisbader H, Kupperman HS. Vitamin E and Climacteric syndrome. *Arch Intern Med* 1953;91:792–9

44. Alder E. The Blatt Kupperman menopausal index: a critique. *Maturitas* 1998;29:19–24

45. WHOQOL Group. The World Health organization quality of life assessment (WHOQOL): development and general psychometric properties. *Soc Sci Med* 1998;46:1569–85

46. Hunt S, McEwen J, McKenna S. Measuring health status: a new tool for clinicians and epidemiologists. *J Royal Coll Gen Pract* 1985;35:185–8

47. Jenkinson C. Comparison of UK and US methods for weighting and scoring the SF36 summary measures. *J Pub Health Med* 1999;21:3270–376

48. Jenkinson C, Stewart Brown S, Paterson S, *et al.* Assessment of the SGF-36 version 2 in the united Kingdom. *J Epidemiol Commun Health* 1999;53:46–50

49. Ledesert B, Ringa V, Breart G. Menopause and perceived health status among the women of the French GAZEL cohort. *Maturitas* 1995;20:113–20

50. Oldenhaave A, Jazmeann LJB, Haspels AA, *et al.* The impact of climacteric on well-being: a survey based on 5213 women 39–60 years old. *Am J Obstet Gynecol* 1993;168:772–80

51. Dennerstein L. Well-being, symptoms and the menopausal transition. *Maturitas* 1996;23:147–57

52. Jacobs PA, Hyland ME, Ley A. Self rated menopausal status and quality of life in women aged 40–63 years. *Br J Health Psychol* 2000;5:395–411

53. Hyland ME, Sodegren SC. Development of a new type of global quality of life scale and the comparison of performance and preference for 12 global scales. *Quality Life Res* 1996;5:469–80

Methodology in studies of the menopausal transition: lessons from observational studies   **2**

L. Dennerstein and J. Guthrie

INTRODUCTION*

There has been much ongoing debate over which symptoms and health outcomes are related to the hormonal aspects of the menopausal transition, and which are pre-existing or relate to aging or other psycho-social factors. Conflicting findings reflect some of the methodological difficulties inherent in studies of the menopause, as well as specific issues pertaining to the measurement of symptoms and quality of life. This chapter examines some of these issues and includes relevant examples from the population-based prospective study of the menopausal transition, the Melbourne Women's Midlife Health Project (MWMHP).

PRINCIPLES OF GOOD PRACTICE IN WOMEN'S HEALTH RESEARCH

Menopause research, like other fields of women's health research, has been criticized in the past for medicalizing women's experiences and treating women as research objects. Applying the principles of good practice in women's health to menopause research will overcome these criticisms and lead to research more able to answer the controversial issues remaining in this field. The principles of good practice in women's health were recently defined in an initiative of the Commonwealth Secretariat[2]. The 1995 Eleventh Commonwealth Health Ministers Meeting on Women and Health recognized that many countries have innovative projects that are sensitively addressing issues of concern to women. A priority recommendation was to collect and disseminate models of good practice on women and health and to give annual Commonwealth Awards for Excellence. The Commonwealth initiative aimed to set standards for good practice in women's health and to profile and thus assist the development of approaches that address the real health disadvantages of women.

The Principles of Good Practice in Women's Health were developed from the growing women's health literature and the platforms of action of the three recent UN conferences on women. The principles were revised after input from a panel of international experts from a range of countries, and presented at several international conferences for further comment. The framework was then piloted in countries with a range of economic development. The principles are broadly based so they could be applied to research, training, evaluation, policy formation and intervention strategies. Table 1 summarizes the principles and the general themes. An individual project will not necessarily include all of these features.

The first set of principles deals with the need for a broad-based scope or focus. The second set acknowledges the multiple determinants of women's health, and thus the need for research projects to measure a broad range of determinants (physical, psychosocial, gender roles and other factors indicating the diversity

---

*This chapter draws heavily on sections of reference 1. Adapted and reprinted with permission of *Quality of Life Research*, Kluwer Academic Publishers, the Netherlands

Table 1 Good practice principles

Scope

1 Women's health concerns extend over the life cycle and are not limited to reproductive problems
2 Women's health problems include, but are not limited to, conditions, diseases or disorders which are specific to women, occur more commonly in women, or have differing risk factors or course in women than in men
3 Health must be considered in broad terms and both positively as well as negatively. Dimensions of health include the physical, mental, social and spiritual

Determinants

4 Women's health is directly affected by a range of socio-cultural, physical and psychological factors
5 Women have gender roles and responsibilities that directly affect their level of access to and control of resources necessary to protect their health. These resources are both external (economic, political, information/education, a safe environment free of violence and time) and internal (self-esteem, initiative)
6 Women are diverse in their age, class, race or ethnicity, religion, functional capacity, sexual orientation and social circumstances. These factors may lead to inequities which adversely affect their health

Community participation

7 Priority should be given to issues that have been identified as important by women themselves. Particular attention should be paid to those issues raised by women who are subject to inequities in their society
8 Women from the target community should be involved in the planning, implementation and evaluation of projects involving their health
9 Knowledge arising from projects must be accessible to all women but particularly women in the target community. This also means that information must be provided in forms appropriate to different levels of education and literacy methods

Methods

10 To address the complex issues affecting women's health a broad-based, interdisciplinary, gendered approach is needed, involving and bringing together the knowledge and methods of social and health scientists and other disciplines where appropriate
11 Intersectoral approaches are needed to address the social factors affecting women's health and life chances. These may involve the working together of various governmental departments, non-governmental and community-based groups and the private sector
12 Knowledge from projects should also inform and influence government policies and plans, legislation, research and healthcare workers
13 Where possible there should be resource-sharing of skills within regions

of women). Research methods need to include interdisciplinary approaches to bring together knowledge from a range of disciplines and appropriate methods for acquiring meaningful data on both determinants and health outcomes. A common theme evident in the UN conference papers and women's health literature is the value of community participation. Consultations or meetings with groups of women can be used to identify the issues that need to be addressed in a research project. Women's groups can also assist with strategies for providing accessible information back to women in the community.

POPULATION STUDY ISSUES

Study type

Clearly there are a number of different research modes which could be used to explore whether the menopausal transition affects quality of life, varying from basic science models, to studies of primates (often involving extirpative surgery and then hormonal intervention), and clinical trials of women who may have reached natural menopause or had menopause induced. However, clinical experience is known to be based on a small proportion of self-selecting, predominantly ill women and may not be representative of most women's experience of the menopause[3,4]. Population-based studies have demonstrated that women who seek treatment differ in systematic ways from those who do not[3,4]. Patient-based samples are biased in terms of education, socio-economic status, other health problems and incidence of general depression[5]. Observational studies that aim to determine the prevalence of health outcomes and factors related to these should utilize a population or community derived sample rather than a clinic sample. Only studies of women derived randomly from the general population provide findings which can be confidently generalized to be the experience of most women of that particular culture and geographic location. Population studies also provide a range of health outcomes to study in real life settings, unlike those of clinical trials in which small samples or entry criteria exclude the possibility of looking at a range of variables that may affect the outcome under study.

The MWMHP sample was found by random telephone digital dialling of phone numbers in the Melbourne urban area of Australia to identify women aged 45–55 years who were Australian-born[6].

Rating scales

Health outcomes and their determinants can be measured by validated rating scales. The failure to use adequately validated scales has been a major problem in menopause research. This particularly applies to the measurement of sexuality and of symptom experience (see below). For example, with regard to sexuality, relatively few of the population-based studies of the menopausal transition have made any inquiry about sexual functioning. Differing measures of sexual functioning have been used with studies often failing to offer any data on the validity or reliability of these measures in their local population. Some of the assessments have been very vague constructs indeed. For example Osborn and colleagues[7] asked a general practice population if they suffered from 'sexual dysfunction' while Koster and

Garde[8] asked women whether sexual desire was decreased or infrequent compared with 11 years previously.

The MWMHP utilized and adapted the McCoy Female Sexuality Questionnaire as the measure of female sexual functioning[9]. The modified scale (Personal Experiences Questionnaire) was then subjected to factor analysis[10] and subsequently shortened using an optimization procedure[11].

The research process itself may result in response bias. This includes interviewer bias in the phrasing of questions, and specification bias if the variable under study is not well specified to the full understanding of the subject.

Measuring symptoms

This area is discussed in detail in Chapter 3. The standard method used for collecting information on the prevalence and severity of symptoms has been a checklist of symptoms. A commonly ignored issue is that the checklist itself introduces a number of biases including the problem of elicitation. Wright[12], interviewing women of the Navajo tribe, found that virtually all respondents reported no bodily changes since menopause in response to open-ended questions but most responded positively to symptoms in the checklist. Holte[13] noted that the sounder the methodology, the lower the prevalence of symptoms. When frequency or bothersomeness of complaint are included, the reporting rate goes down further[13]. For example, irritability was reported by 57% of premenopausal women as being present occasionally but by 10% of premenopausal women as being present frequently. The occasional presence of symptoms does not indicate their impact on the woman and is not clinically relevant or indicative of treatment needs.

The MWMHP used a 33 item symptom check list in which women were asked to indicate whether they had been bothered by any of the symptoms listed in the prior two weeks[14]. Each symptom was scored on a four-point scale in terms of severity. Utilizing data from the first seven years of follow-up, the

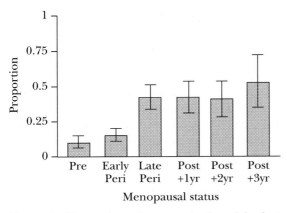

Figure 1 Proportion of women bothered by hot flushes. Pre, premenopausal; Early Peri, change in menstrual frequency; Late Peri, 3–11 months amenorrhea; Post +1 yr, 12–23 months amenorrhea; Post +2 yr, 24–35 months amenorrhea; Post +3 yr ≥ 36 months amenorrhea. Reproduced with permission, *Obstetrics and Gynecology*[14]

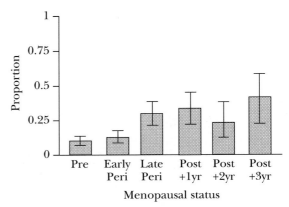

Figure 2 Proportion of women bothered by night sweats. Pre, premenopausal; Early Peri, change in menstrual frequency; Late Peri, 3–11 months amenorrhea; Post +1 yr, 12–23 months amenorrhea; Post +2 yr, 24–35 months amenorrhea; Post +3 yr ≥ 36 months amenorrhea. Reproduced with permission, *Obstetrics and Gynecology*[14]

means of symptom severity over the early phase of the menopausal transition were compared with those from the later part of the menopausal transition when women had experienced three months or more of amenorrhea or had become postmenopausal. Increasing from early to late menopausal transition were the number of women reporting: five or more symptoms (+14%), hot flushes (+27%), night sweats (+17%) and dry vagina (+17%) (all $p < 0.05$). Breast soreness/ tenderness decreased with the menopausal transition (–21%). Trouble with sleeping increased by +6%. The major change in prevalence occurred from early to late menopausal transition, except for insomnia which showed a gradual increase (see Figures 1–5). It should be noted that many of the symptom scales used in climacteric research do not include some of the key symptoms (breast tenderness, vaginal dryness, dyspareunia) shown to change dramatically with the menopausal transition.

Role of culture

McKinlay and McKinlay[15] commented on the presence of inter- and intracultural differences in symptom reporting: "a physiological

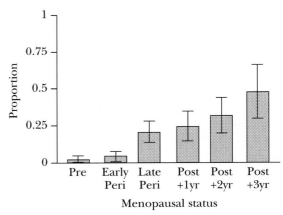

Figure 3 Proportion of women bothered by dryness of vagina. Pre, premenopausal; Early Peri, change in menstrual frequency; Late Peri, 3–11 months amenorrhea; Post +1 yr, 12–23 months amenorrhea; Post +2 years, 24–35 months amenorrhea; Post +3 yr ≥ 36 months amenorrhea. Reproduced with permission, *Obstetrics and Gynecology*[14]

condition may not necessarily be the subject of complaint". Kaufert and Syrotuik[16] also described how stereotypes held by different social and cultural groups act as a framework, within which an individual can select, organize and label experience. In menopause research

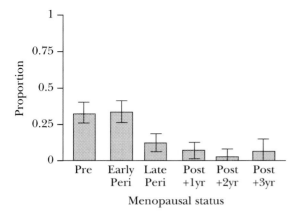

Figure 4 Proportion of women bothered by breast soreness. Pre, premenopausal; Early Peri, change in menstrual frequency; Late Peri, 3–11 months amenorrhea; Post +1 yr, 12–23 months amenorrhea; Post +2 yr, 24–35 months amenorrhoea; Post +3 yr ≥ 36 months amenorrhea. Reproduced with permission, *Obstetrics and Gynecology*[14]

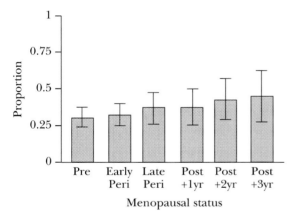

Figure 5 Proportion of women bothered by trouble sleeping. Pre, premenopausal; Early Peri, change in menstrual frequency; Late Peri, 3–11 months amenorrhea; Post +1 yr, 12–23 months amenorrhea; Post +2 yr, 24–35 months amenorrhea; Post +3 yr ≥ 36 months amenorrhea. Reproduced with permission, *Obstetrics and Gynecology*[14]

there is a risk that stereotypes will become operative whenever subjects know the topic of the research. In order to minimize bias due to stereotypes held about menopause, Kaufert and Syrotuik[16] did not use the word menopause in the title of the questionnaire and they placed the symptom checklist in a section on general health. This general recommendation has been followed by a number of later studies of women's experience of the menopausal transition[3,6].

The title of the Melbourne Women's Midlife Health Project was similarly chosen so as not to elicit underlying societal stereotypes of the relationship of menopause to health[6]. The findings of the MWMHP are based on a Caucasian sample.

Measures of ovarian function

Menopausal status

The time of change for a woman approaching the end of her reproductive life can be conceptualised from an endocrine perspective as "the period of maximum hormonal fluctuation preceding final menses"[17], but no single biochemical measurement is acceptable as a defining marker of where this phase begins or ends. It is the outward sign of hormonal change through a woman's menstrual status that has gained acceptance as the most useful measure of a woman's ovarian status[17].

In 1985 the Korpilampi workshop[18] focused on the problems and issues relating to the definition of menopausal status. At the time of this workshop, the criteria used to define the boundary between the pre- and perimenopausal states included the reporting of changes in menstrual flow and/or regularity. The workshop identified that the reliability of such definitions for predicting the further movement to postmenopause had not been sufficiently studied. They concluded that more research was necessary to define the onset of the perimenopause, particularly by linking together analyses of hormone levels with self-reported changes in menstrual patterns and symptom experience[18].

The MWMHP[6,19] followed a population-based sample of 438 mid-aged women through the menopausal transition, collecting annual data on menstrual histories including changes in menstrual frequency (regularity), menstrual flow and episodes of amenorrhea. These data were analysed longitudinally to determine which aspects of menstrual change best predict time to becoming postmenopausal[17]. Three months of amenorrhea was found to be the best predictor of future menopause, followed by changes in menstrual frequency. Change in flow only was not predictive of future menopause. Analysis of menstrual diary data from the MWMHP by Taffe and Dennerstein[20] found that there was poor reliability for women's annual self-reports of change in menstrual frequency and flow. Based on these findings a two-stage classification scheme is suggested for defining the menopausal transition: 'early' for mid-aged women who may or may not report menstrual irregularities but without two skipped periods, and 'late' defined as the self-report of 3–11 months of amenorrhea. This recommendation is in accord with those of the 2001 STRAW Workshop, Park City[21].

Hormone measures

Relatively few studies have undertaken any hormonal determinations. Studies of the role of menopausal status seem to be based on the hypothesis that any changes in health outcomes reflecting the menopause will be evident in postmenopausal women having different levels of the variable under study to women who have not reached menopause (defined as 12 months of amenorrhea). Yet endocrine change occurs for some years prior to cessation of menopause[22], so it would seem important to acquire measures of all variables while women are still menstruating regularly, some years before menses cease. Other issues involved in hormone measures have been those of the frequency of sampling (annual versus daily or weekly), type of sampling (plasma, urine, salivary), phase of the cycle sampled and the presence of floor effects, due to the lack of sensitivity of assays at the lower levels of estradiol and inhibin that occur in the postmenopause.

The MWMHP found that 63% of estradiol values were below the level of sensitivity of the assay (20 pmol/l) when women were 12 months or more after the final menstrual period.

Age and length of follow-up

Age at baseline and length of follow-up are important issues. Follow-up has often been only in the order of three years[23–25]. The MWMHP found that after three years of follow-up, only 12% of women had become naturally postmenopausal (12 months of no bleeding after reaching final menstrual period). At the end of seven years of follow-up only 39% of the women in this cohort were naturally postmenopausal, reflecting splintering of the sample as well as length of follow-up (Figure 6)

Natural menopausal transition versus induced menopause

A major problem in menopause research has been to establish the health experiences associated with the natural menopausal experience and how these may differ when menopause is induced. A number of studies suggest that symptom experience is likely to be worse when women have undergone surgical menopause[3]. Documentation of medical treatment that may impact on ovarian functioning (surgery, chemotherapy, irradiation) and documentation of medication taken by women is needed so that these women may be treated separately in the analysis.

Exogenous hormones

Exogenous hormones may mask the effects of changing ovarian function, so women taking the oral contraceptive pill or any sort of hormone therapy must also be treated separately in analyses. In many countries an increasing number of women are choosing to adopt hormone therapy, and this may lead to a splintering of the sample and even to insufficient numbers to examine the effects of the natural menopausal transition. Holte[26] reported that sample size in a longitudinal study over five years was reduced from 200 to 56.

Prospective studies allow the profile of those who take up hormone therapy to be compared with that of non-users so that any biases related to hormone selection and which may affect the

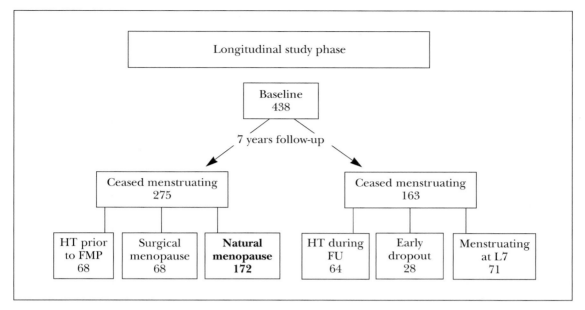

Figure 6 Attrition from Melbourne Women's Midlife Health Project. HT, hormone treatment; FU, follow-up; FMP, final menstrual period; L7, seventh year of follow-up (reproduced with permission, *Qual Life Res* 2000;9:721–31[1])

end-point can be established. Guthrie and colleagues[27] found that hormone therapy users did not differ significantly from non-users in lifestyle, sociodemographic and cardiovascular risk factors or in most health status factors, prior to taking hormone therapy. Hormone therapy users were significantly more likely to report a history of premenstrual complaints; to have had a breast examination by a health professional; to agree that women 'regret when their period stops for the last time'; to report that they took non-prescription medications; and to have had a tubal ligation.

Cross-sectional versus longitudinal design

Population-based studies often suffer from being cross-sectional in design[28], rather than having the power of longitudinal analysis of the same women through the menopausal transition[29]. Cross-sectional studies can only indicate whether associations exist and are unable to determine the direction of causality. But cross-sectional studies do have certain advantages. For a start, they are more convenient and less expensive to carry out.

Subjects are only asked to participate on one occasion, and so the response rate is likely to be higher than when subjects are asked to contribute time for assessments on a regular basis. Those who agree to participate in a longitudinal study may differ in certain systematic ways from those who decline and this may introduce bias into the study sample population[19]. Thus the sample participating in a cross-sectional study may be more similar to a general population sample than that of a longitudinal study sample. Splintering of the study population can continue for other reasons during the accrual process[30]. From the target group only those persons available to the investigator are potentially eligible for study. Further splintering occurs after applying inclusion and exclusion criteria. Even after being admitted to the study the subject's records must be properly filled in: missing data on some variables can lead to exclusion of the subject with some analytic techniques. If the reason for drop-out or premature early termination of the study is related to the studied end-point, this can induce further bias.

Another source of error is that of con-

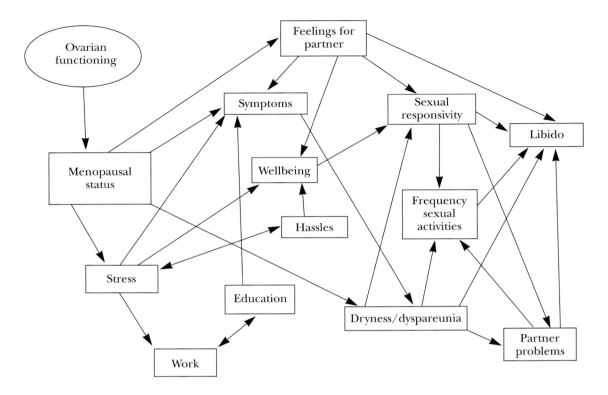

Figure 7 Model of factors affecting sexual functioning (reproduced with permission, *Climacteric* 1999;2: 254–62[33])

founding, which necessitates the need for multivariate analytic methods to control for the influence of the various factors that can affect an outcome. The majority of community based studies have been cross-sectional and thus limit researchers to inferring apparent associations. Cross-sectional studies cannot control for premenopausal characteristics nor separate the effects of aging from those of menopause. These studies are less satisfactory than longitudinal studies in which the same women are being followed over time with the same instruments, so that what is being observed is change in the same population with time.

Longitudinal cohort designs facilitate the identification of those associations most likely to reflect a cause–effect relationship and separate the effects of aging from those of menopause[5]. But most longitudinal studies have used inadequate statistical methods, often resorting to a cross-sectional approach to

data which, as repeated measures, are no longer independent in nature[31]. Longitudinal collection of data reduces reliance on memory for long recall periods. The length of the recall period in cross-sectional studies can lead to further inaccuracy of data. This is not only true for the studied end-points, but also for possible covariates at the time of occurrence. In longitudinal studies there is the opportunity for measures to be made prospectively (such as menstrual diaries) rather than relying on self-recall, which may be substantially less accurate[20]. When change over time is the key concern, a prospective design is mandatory.

The longitudinal nature of the MWMHP established the importance of baseline characteristics in predicting later mood. For example, the most important predictor of positive mood at postmenopause was positive mood score at baseline while women were still in the early part of the menopausal transition[32].

Statistical analysis

Most studies have utilised only univariate analysis and thus been unable to take into account the role of confounding or interacting factors. Hence the findings of these studies are often contradictory. A major problem for longitudinal studies has been the lack of a sufficiently sensitive statistical analysis that would use a 'within subject repeated measures' method, allowing for the various factors that may affect the quality of life measure, changes in those factors and interactions with the menopausal transition[31].

The analysis of longitudinal studies becomes more complex as the temporal dimension is added to the other possible components of the study. Many statistical approaches are possible. To illustrate the diversity of the possible approaches, Lehert and Dennerstein[31] carried out a literature search on past analyses of longitudinal studies. Concentrating on the keywords 'cohorts', 'longitudinal series', 'time series analysis' and 'panel', they collected 123 papers that were then scrutinised on the particular statistical technique utilised. Four main categories of techniques were found: cross-sectional reduction of data (56%); multifactorial techniques (26%); repeated measurement analysis of variance (14%); and other (time series and structural equation modelling) (4%).

Cross-sectional reduction often violates underlying statistical assumptions. A simple but powerful technique is to calculate mean values prior to and following an event such as the final menstrual period. Linear regression is preferred to logistic regression where continuous data are available, to allow for the influence of multiple factors. When more information about changes over time is required, more complex techniques are needed: a suitable technique is 'repeated measures multivariate analysis of variance', using several contrasts to estimate various effects. Simple split plot or randomized block designs are not recommended as they often violate compound symmetry assumptions. For series involving more than 100 observations for each subject, time series and spectral analysis techniques should be considered. Structural equation modeling is recommended for detailed examination of factors that may influenced both the studied endpoint, and the presence of feedback and of latent or non-measurable variable[31].

An example of structural equation modeling is given in Figure 7, reprinted from Dennerstein et al[33]. This modeling allows the various factors influencing aspects of sexual functioning to be depicted as well as the relationships of the different aspects of sexual functioning to each other. The strength of each equation depicted is given separately as regression coefficients.

Recommendations

Several strategies have been suggested to overcome problems in study design. These include describing the study as a general health survey, so that bias caused by emotional response to menopause is lessened; collecting information on current symptomatology so that the problem of recall bias is minimized; utilizing an age range that encompasses the menopausal transition i.e. 40–55 years for cross-sectional studies, or a younger age group for longitudinal studies of the menopausal transition to ensure that women are premenopausal at outset; longer follow-up in longitudinal studies; and collection of prospective data on menstruation and any hormone usage so that the phase of menopausal transition can be adequately determined.

References

1. Dennerstein L, Helmes E. The menopausal transition and quality of life: methodologic issues. *Qual Life Res* 2000;9:721–31
2. Commonwealth Secretariat. *Models of Good Practice Relevant to Women and Health.* London, 1997
3. McKinlay J,. McKinlay S, Brambilla D. Health status and utilization behavior associated with menopause. *Am J Epidemiol* 1987;125:110–21
4. Morse C, Smith A, Dennerstein L, *et al.* The treatment-seeking woman at menopause. *Maturitas* 1994;18:161–73
5. Avis N, McKinlay S. The Massachusetts Women's Health Study: an epidemiologic investigation of the menopause. *J Am Med Womens Assoc* 1995;50:45–9,63
6. Dennerstein L, Smith A, Morse C, *et al.* Menopausal symptoms in Australian women. *Med J Austr* 1993;159:232–6
7. Osborn M, Hawton K, Gath D. Sexual dysfunction among middle aged women in the community. *Br Med J* 1988;296:959–62
8. Koster A, Garde K. Sexual desire and menopausal development. A prospective study of Danish women born in 1936. *Maturitas* 1993;16:49–60
9. McCoy NL, Matyas JR. Oral contraceptives and sexuality in university women. *Arch Sex Behav* 1996;25:73–90
10. Dennerstein L, Dudley E, Hopper J, *et al.* Sexuality, hormones and the menopausal transition. *Maturitas* 1997;26:83–93
11. Dennerstein L, Lehert P, Dudley E. Short scale to measure female sexuality: adapted from McCoy Female Sexuality questionnaire. *J Sex Marital Therapy* 2001;27:339–51
12. Wright, A. On the calculation of climacteric symptoms. *Maturitas* 1981;3:55–63
13. Holte, A. Prevalence of climacteric complaints in a representative sample of middle-aged women in Oslo, Norway. *J Psychosom Obstet Gynecol* 1991;303–17
14. Dennerstein L, Dudley EC, Hopper JL, *et al.* A prospective population-based study of menopausal symptoms. *Obstet Gynecol* 2000;96:351–8
15. McKinlay, SM, McKinlay JB. Selected studies of the menopause – a methodological critique. *J Biol Sci* 1973;5:533–55
16. Kaufert P, Syrotuik J. Symptom reporting at the menopause. *Soc Sci Med E* 1981;15:173–84
17. Dudley E, Hopper J, Taffe J, *et al.* Using longitudinal data to define the perimenopause by menstrual cycle characteristics. *Climacteric* 1998; 1:18–25
18. Kaufert P, Lock M, McKinlay S, *et al.* Menopause Research: The Korpilampi Workshop. *Soc Sci Med* 1986;22:1285–9
19. Burger H, Dudley E, Hopper J, *et al.* The endocrinology of the menopausal transition: a cross-sectional study of a population-based sample. *J Clin Endocrinol Metab* 1995;30:12: 3537–45
20. Taffe J, Dennerstein L. Retrospective self-report compared with menstrual diary data prospectively kept during the menopausal transition. *Climacteric* 2000;3:183–91
21. Soules MR, Shermans S, Parrott E, *et al.* Executive summary: Stages of Reproductive Aging Workshop (STRAW). *Fertil Steril* 2001;76:874–8
22. Burger H, Dudley E, Groome N, *et al.* Prospectively measured changes of serum FSH, estradiol, and the dimeric inhibins during the menopausal transition in a population-based cohort of women. *J Clin Endocrinol Metab* 1999; 84:4025–30
23. Kaufert P, Gilbert P, Tate R. The Manitoba Project: a re-examination of the link between menopause and depression. *Maturitas* 1992;14: 143–55
24. Bromberger J, Matthews K. A longitudinal study of the effects of pessimism, trait anxiety, and life stress on depressive symptoms in middle aged women. *Psychol Aging* 1996;11:207–13
25. Woods N, Mitchell E. Patterns of depressed mood in midlife women; observations from the Seattle Midlife Women's Health Study. *Res Nurs Health* 1996;19:111–23
26. Holte, A. Influences of natural menopause on health complaints: a prospective study of healthy Norwegian women. *Maturitas* 1992;14: 127–41
27. Guthrie J, Garamszegi C, Dudley E, *et al.* Hormone therapy use in Australian-born women: a longitudinal study. *Med J Aust* 1999; 171:358–61
28. Van Keep P, Kellerhals J. The ageing woman. About the influence of some social and cultural factors on the changes in attitude and behaviour that occur during and after the menopause. *Acta Obstet Gynecol Scand Suppl* 1976;51:17–27

29. McCoy N, Davidson J. A longitudinal study of the effects of menopause on sexuality. *Maturitas* 1985;7:203–10

30. Wheeler J. A multivariate look at the menopause. *J Clin Epidemiol* 1989;42:1029–30

31. Lehert P, Dennerstein L. Statistical techniques for the analysis of change in longitudinal studies of the menopause. *Acta Obstet Gynecol* 2001, in press

32. Dennerstein L, Lehert P, Dudley E, *et al.* Factors contributing to positive mood during the menopausal transition. *J Nerv Ment Dis* 2000: 189:84–9

33. Dennerstein L, Lehert P, Burger H, *et al.* Factors affecting sexual functioning of women in the midlife years. *Climacteric* 1999;2:254–62

Measuring the symptom dimension of quality of life: general and menopause-specific scales and their subscale structure

3

J. G. Greene

INTRODUCTION

In the context of health, quality of life (QoL) refers to the impact ill health has on various aspects of an individual's life situation and circumstances. Measures of QoL, therefore, generally attempt to gauge the effect ill health has across a number of physical, psychological and social parameters. For example, the widely used QoL measure, the SF-36, evaluates in all eight different dimensions of QoL[1]. These include physical functioning, role functioning, social functioning, vitality and so on. Like many such measures of QoL, it also contains a measure of mental health, assessed in the form of psychological symptoms.

This chapter will largely focus on the last named of the various dimensions of QoL of climacteric women, namely their symptomatology, in the course of which, the principles and rationale underlying methods of assessing the numerous symptoms of which many women complain at that time of their lives will be outlined.

This will culminate in the final and main section of this chapter, in which current standardized menopause-specific scales will be reviewed.

However, we begin by discussing and defining the concept central to this chapter, namely symptoms.

SYMPTOMS

According to the *Oxford Medical Dictionary*[2] symptoms are:

"An indication of a disease or a disorder noticed by the patient himself. A presenting symptom is one that leads a patient to consult a doctor."

The first part of this definition indicates that symptoms are subjective expressions or manifestations of some underlying physical, psychological or social dysfunction. They are, in effect, evidence of *dis*-ease. There is little doubt that in addition to estrogen-related vasomotor symptoms, many women during the menopause transition – and particularly those presenting at menopause clinics – are experiencing such dysfunction, which manifests itself in the form of a plethora of somatic, psychosomatic and psychological symptoms, sometimes referred to as the 'climacteric syndrome'[3]. Both cross-sectional[4] and longitudinal psychosocial surveys[5–11] of general population samples of climacteric women have shown such symptoms to be associated with a variety of psychosocial problems within the woman's life situations. Table 1 summarizes the sort of psychosocial problems found to be related to depressive symptoms in seven longitudinal studies.

The second part of the above definition emphasizes the part played by symptoms in prompting individuals to seek help. Symptoms initiate doctor–patient contact. In general, individuals do not initially come to clinics or hospitals complaining about underlying physical, psychological or social dysfunction. It

Table 1 Summary of the psychosocial findings of longitudinal studies

Senior author	Country	Factors associated with depression
Holte (1992)[5]	Norway	Poor social network, negative life events
Hunter (1992)[6]	UK	Family problems, bereavement, ill-health, negative attitudes
Kaufert (1992)[7]	Canada	Domestic problems, poor health
Avis (1994)[8]	USA	Illness, death of family members, negative attitudes, perceived health status
Dennerstein (1994)[9]	Australia	Interpersonal problems, attitude to aging, current health status, life style
Collins (1995)[10]	Sweden	Living alone, life style
Woods (1996)[11]	USA	Stressful life events, negative attitudes, health status

is the subjective experience of this dysfunction, in the form of symptoms, of which they complain. Furthermore, symptoms are important as a measure of outcome of treatment, since symptom relief is evidence that the treatment has been successful in resolving the underlying dysfunction. It is for these reasons that symptoms are important and their reliable and valid measurement essential.

Reliable and valid measures of multi-symptom conditions generally come in the form of scales and subscales, developed on the basis of principles of test construction and scaling[12]. Issues relating to scales and subscales will be discussed in the following section of this chapter.

SCALES AND SUBSCALES

Objective and consistent measurement of phenomena within its sphere of interest is the foundation of all scientific investigation, whether it be in sociology or nuclear physics. Without this foundation little progress can be made. In the field of psychology the techniques developed to construct such measures became known as psychometrics. Psychometrics has its roots in the first experimental psychology laboratory founded by Wilhelm Wundt at the University of Leipzig in 1870. Initially, interest focused on establishing general principles underlying such phenomena as human sensation, perception, memory and learning and so on. However, the subjects

under investigation invariably showed wide variation on these tasks leading to the development of interest in individual differences. The assessment of differences between individuals required the construction of measures sensitive enough to distinguish between subjects on the various parameters under investigation. This in turn led to attempts to construct 'scales'. Scales, by definition, are instruments which measure phenomena on a continuum using ordinal scaling. Thus scales give a graded measure of the phenomenon, of supposedly equal intervals, on which individuals can be placed. A tape measure, measuring height, is an example of an equal interval graded scale.

Scales measuring more complex human characteristics, such as intelligence or personality traits, invariably consist of a *number* of items which are summated to give an overall score for each person. Scales designed to assess conditions of multiple symptomatology, are also of this nature. That is, they consist of a number of symptoms, yielding a total score which reflects the degree of severity of the condition along a graded continuum for each individual. In addition, each symptom is usually rated in terms of its frequency of occurrence or severity. This is a more sensitive way of measuring the person's experience of the symptoms rather than crude rating of present/absent, which gives no indication of the magnitude of the person's experience of the symptom or degree of suffering.

Scales measuring complex phenomena or syndromes, which may have many facets, are generally made up of a number of *subscales*, each measuring a different facet of the syndrome. The practice of summating symptoms from demonstrably different domains is often meaningless. It is like adding a person's height and waist measurements to give an overall measure of 'size'. Such a measure fails to distinguish tall thin people from small obese people, since both would tend to have a similar overall 'size' score. The opposite and common practice of reporting findings for symptoms individually is also unacceptable, since such a measure tends to be insensitive and unstable and fails to comprehensively assess the condition.

Scales measuring human characteristics or conditions can be categorized into two types, general scales and condition-specific scales. The former are scales which have been developed for general use and can be used to measure characteristics across different conditions. The latter are designed specifically for use with an identified condition group.

For many decades there existed only one menopause-specific scale, the Kuppermann Index[13]. This scale has been used in climacteric research since the 1950s and is still in use, although by a dwindling number of researchers. The reason for its declining use is that it suffers from several inherent psychometric problems: no rationale is provided for the eleven symptoms making up the scale; the symptoms are each assigned an arbitrary weighting; most damaging of all, symptom scores are summated to yield an overall score. This overall score is therefore contributed to by symptoms from different domains – vasomotor, somatic and psychological. Because of its unsound psychometric properties this measure is now seriously discredited and should be discarded[14].

GENERAL SYMPTOM SCALES IN CLIMACTERIC RESEARCH

The term general scales, in the present context, refers to measures that have been constructed on populations other than climacteric women. They are designed for general use. That is, they can be used to assess symptomatology in different populations, either clinical samples or general population samples. For example, a scale such as the Beck Depression Index[15], although constructed using psychiatric patients, can be used to assess the degree of clinical depression in patients attending general hospitals, in general practice samples or among the general population. The general scales that have been most commonly used in climacteric research are the General Health Questionnaire[16,17], the Hamilton Rating Scales of Clinical Anxiety and Depression[18,19], the Beck Depression Index[16,17,20,21], the Zung Anxiety Scale[22], the Kellner–Sheffield scale[22] and the Centre for Epidemiologic Studies Depression Scale (CES-D)[23]. The CES-D Scale, a measure developed specifically to assess depression in epidemiological studies of general populations[24], has been used in the previously referenced large scale longitudinal studies of the climacteric carried out in North America: the Manitoba Project[7], the Massachusetts Women's Health Study[8], and the Seattle Midlife Women's Health Study[1].

Usually researchers will use more than one scale in their investigations and several of the foregoing scales also contain subscales measuring different aspects of mental health. For example the General Health Questionnaire contains four subscales, the Hamilton Scale two and the Kellner–Sheffield four.

Although the general scales used in climacteric research have been shown to be reliable and valid symptom measures, care must be exercised in their use and interpretation with populations on which they have not been standardized, particularly patient groups with medical conditions. The main problem is that many of them contain symptoms known as vegetative symptoms or somatic symptoms. For example, a symptom such as loss of appetite can be a symptom of psychiatric depression, but it can also be a symptom of many medical conditions. The result is that scales, developed for use with psychiatric patients, may exaggerate the degree of psychopathology among patients with medical conditions. In the context of climacteric research, a good example of this exaggeration relates to the General Health Questionnaire. This scale contains one item on hot flushes, one on sweating and six relating to sleep, a complaint which in climacteric women is often thought to be due to night sweats. It is no surprise therefore that the indiscriminate use of the General Health Questionnaire to detect 'psychiatric cases' among perimenopausal women in the general population produces a spuriously high psychiatric morbidity rate of 47% in that group[25]. Furthermore, the depressed mood shown by climacteric women is not only less severe than that of psychiatric patients but it may have different origins and may have a different symptom picture than psychiatric depression. For example, it has been shown in two clinical trials of hormone replacement therapy that the Beck Depression Index, which was designed to assess clinical depression in psychiatric patients, was much less sensitive to change than were other non-psychiatric measures[16,20]. This was because on that Index the mean score of climacteric women in both trials was so low that they came within the non-clinically depressed category, thus leaving little scope for change or improvement.

In recent years a number of climacteric-specific scales, based on a long-standing psychometric method of scale construction, have been developed. That method is the mathematical technique of factor analysis. These climacteric-specific scales will be reviewed in the final section of this chapter but before doing so it is necessary to describe the principles and rationale underlying factor analysis.

PRINCIPLES AND RATIONALE OF FACTOR ANALYSIS

Factor analysis is a multi-variant mathematical technique traditionally used in psychometrics to construct measures of psychological and behavioral characteristics, such as intellectual abilities or personality traits. From a theoretical standpoint it addresses the problems of analyzing the structure of the inter-

relationships (correlations) among a large number of variables (test scores, questionnaire responses, behaviors, symptoms) by identifying a set of underlying dimensions known as factors. The overall objective of factor analysis is data summarization and data reduction.

In summarizing the data, factor analysis derives underlying dimensions that, when interpreted and understood, describe the data using much fewer dimensions than original variables. Data reduction is achieved by calculating scores for each of the underlying dimensions and substituting them for the many original individual variable scores. A central aim of factor analysis is the orderly simplification of a number of interrelated measures. Factor analysis seeks to do precisely what humans have been engaged in throughout history, namely to make order out of the apparent chaos of their environment. Factor analysis, like all scientific endeavors, aims to order and give structure to observed variables. It also has a direct practical application in that on the basis of that order and structure, measuring instruments can be constructed in the form of scales and subscales.

Factor analysis was first used in psychometrics by the British psychologist Charles Spearman[26] to investigate the structure of human intelligence. By intercorrelating a number of tasks of ability Spearman identified a large general factor, which became known as 'intelligence', running throughout these tasks, and a number of smaller factors representing 'specific' abilities. This became known as the Two-Factor Theory of human ability. Factor analysis was later used by personality theorists to investigate the structure of human personality in the same way, and to develop measures of different personality traits[27,28].

Finally, it was used by psychologists and psychiatrists to investigate the structure of complex psychiatric syndromes and to develop symptom scales to assess different aspects of these syndromes[29,30]. In this context, the technique involves analyzing the intercorrelations among large numbers of symptoms, and factor analyzing the resultant intercorrelation matrix to identify which symptoms cluster together to form groups or factors –

Table 2 Subscale structure of each standardized menopause-specific scale

Greene Climacteric Scale	Women's Health Questionnaire	Menopausal Symptom List	Menopause Rating Scale	Utian QoL Score
Vasomotor	Vasomotor	Vasosomatic	Somatovegetative	Emotional
Somatic	Somatic	General Somatic	Urogenital	Occupational
Anxiety	Anxiety	Psychological	Psychological	Health
Depression	Depression			Sexual
	Cognitive			
	Sleep			
	Sex			
	Menstrual			

data summarization. This allows one to delineate the different facets of the symptom picture and to identify those symptoms which are an essential part of the syndrome picture and those which are not – data reduction. The relationship between a symptom and a factor is measured by a correlation coefficient, known as a factor loading. It is then possible to construct an instrument, consisting of several separate subscales, to measure different aspects of the symptom picture, based on the way symptoms cluster together within factors and on the size of their factor loadings. This results in a scale that yields a symptom profile for each subject.

The use of factor analysis is therefore an essential first step in the development of an instrument designed to assess the structure of any condition that presents with a range of multi-faceted symptomatology, such as the climacteric[31,32]. This chapter concludes therefore with a review of current menopause-specific scales that have been constructed on the basis of factor analysis, and that consist of subscales measuring different aspects of climacteric symptomatology.

STANDARDIZED MENOPAUSE-SPECIFIC SCALES

The lack of a standardized menopause-specific instrument to measure the symptoms of climacteric women has long been recognized. The problem was highlighted by Jaszman[33] at the Fourth International Congress on the Menopause in 1984 and later by Utian[34] at the Sixth Congress in 1990. Within the last decade the situation has dramatically changed. There are now currently available, to the author's knowledge, at least five standardized menopause-specific scales – that is, measures which satisfy the following criteria:

(1) They have been constructed on the basis of a factor analysis;

(2) They consist of several subscales, each measuring a different aspect of climacteric symptomatology;

(3) They possess sound psychometric properties; and

(4) They have been standardized using populations of climacteric women.

Each of the five scales reviewed in this section fulfills these four criteria and each consists of a number of subscales corresponding to the factors that have emerged in the course of the factor analysis. The subscale structures for each scale are shown in Table 2 for comparative purposes. The five scales to be reviewed in chronological order of their construction are:

The Greene Climacteric Scale
The Women's Health Questionnaire
The Menopausal Symptom List
The Menopause Rating Scale
The Utian Quality of Life Score

The last named is not exclusively a measure of symptoms, but as the name indicates, measures other aspects of quality of life. It has been included in this review as it fulfills the above

Table 3 Characteristics of each standardized menopause-specific scale

Name of scale	Number of items	Rating points	Rating measure	Number of subscales	Reliability of subscales
Greene Climacteric Scale	21	4	Severity	4	0.83–0.87
Women's Health Questionnaire	32	2	Present/absent	8	0.78–0.96
Menopausal Symptom List	25	6	Frequency Severity	3	0.73–0.83
Menopause Rating Scale	11	5	Severity	3	0.74–0.82[35]
Utian QoL Score	23	5	Severity	4	Not available

four criteria and one of the subscales is in fact a measure of symptoms. Salient details of each of the five scales and their construction are shown in Table 3.

The Greene Climacteric Scale

This was the first climacteric symptom scale to have been constructed on the basis of a factor analysis. Forty symptoms presented by a group of women attending a menopause clinic were subjected to a principal factor analysis and rotated to oblique structure by the direct Oblimin method[36]. The initial scale consisted of three subscales – vasomotor, somatic and psychological[37].

The subscale structure and symptom content were later modified in the light of the findings of six subsequent factor analytic studies of symptoms presented by climacteric women[38]. Five of the symptoms of the original scale were removed and replaced by four others on the basis of a high consensus across these six studies. The psychological subscale was subdivided into one of anxiety and one of depression for the same reasons, thereby generating four subscales. The final version of the scale consists of 21 symptoms, each rated on a four-point scale of severity. The wording of symptoms was standardized in accordance with the common usage across the seven factorial studies. Test–retest reliability coefficients of the subscales achieve a satisfactory level and over the years of usage the scale has attained a degree of construct validity[38,39].

The Women's Health Questionnaire

This questionnaire was constructed on the basis of a principal component factor analysis with varimax rotation of 36 symptoms reported by a general population sample of climacteric women in south-east England[40]. The final questionnaire consists of eight subscales[41], four of which are identical to those of the Greene Climacteric Scale. The four other subscales – cognitive difficulties, sexual behavior, sleep problems and menstrual symptoms – can be termed 'specific' factors which tend to emerge when a few symptoms relating to a circumscribed complaint are included in the factor analysis. The final scale contains 32 symptoms each rated on a binary scale (0/1). Reliability of the subscales using the test–retest method is satisfactory and concurrent validity has been established for the depressed mood subscale, using the General Health Questionnaire as a comparative measure. Construct validity of the questionnaire has and is being established within a number of current applications. Normative data exist for a wide age range of women[41].

The Menopausal Symptom List

This scale was constructed on the basis of a principal components factor analysis, rotated to oblique structure using the varimax method, of 56 symptoms presented by a small general population of Australian women[43]. The scale consists of three subscales: vasosomatic, general somatic and psychological.

The last named is a combination of the anxiety and depression subscales of the Greene Climacteric Scale and the Women's Health Questionnaire. Unlike these two scales the vasomotor subscale is not a 'pure' measure of vasomotor symptoms but contains other somatic symptoms. The reason for this is not clear, but it may be because the sample was both small and came from a general population. In such a sample the number of women having climacteric-related hot flushes and sweating would be small, and therefore these symptoms would become submerged by other somatic symptoms in the factor analytic procedure.

The final scale contains 25 symptoms, each rated on a six-point scale of both frequency and severity. Test–retest reliability coefficients for all three subscales are satisfactory. Concurrent validity using the Greene Climacteric Scale as a comparative measure was high for the psychological and vasomotor subscales but less so for the general somatic subscale although the correlation did achieve statistical sigmficance[33].

The Menopause Rating Scale

This scale was standardized on a large general population sample of German women, in the course of which a factor analysis identified three independent factors[44]. The scale therefore consists of three subscales psychological, somatovegetative and urogenital. The somato-vegetative subscale contains vasomotor symptoms, in addition to other somatic complaints. The psychological subscale is a combination of anxiety and depressive symptoms.

The final scale consists of 11 symptoms, each rated on a five-point scale of severity. All three subscales and total scores have been shown to have a high degree of stability in a subsample of women followed-up over a one-and-a-half-year period[44]. Both the psychological and somatovegetative subscales were compared with each of the eight domains of the SF-36[44]. While these subscales did not correlate equally well across all dimensions of the SF-36, the pattern of correlations were as would be predicted, with the highest correlations being with those domains of the

SF-36 that are most relevant to women during the menopausal transition.

The Utian Menopause Quality of Life Score

This scale was based on a two-stage factorial process. First, an exploratory principal component analysis was carried out, followed by a factor analysis using a promax rotation of 40 symptoms presented by a sample of women, recruited from obstetric/gynecological practices and hospital employees in the east and midwest USA[46]. These procedures yielded four factors. As the name indicates, the scale is not exclusively a symptom measure, although it does contain one scale relating to emotional well-being. The other subscales measure the effect the menopause transition may have on occupational, health and sexual aspects of QoL.

The final scale consists of 23 items, each rated on a five-point Likert scale. As this is a scale that has only recently been developed, reliability and validity data are not as yet available, although internal consistency of the scale has been demonstrated using the Cronbach method of Alpha analysis. The authors advocate their scale should be used in conjunction with a standardized measure of climacteric symptoms.

CONCLUSION

There now exists a selection of menopause-specific scales, all standardized on samples of climacteric women, all factorially valid, all having a subscale structure and all with sound psychometric properties. It is therefore no longer acceptable for clinicians and researchers to make use of *ad hoc* measures and other measures with poor psychometric properties.

Additionally, researchers have at their disposal a number of standardized general scales that also have satisfactory psychometric properties, but as these have been standardized on populations other than climacteric women, care must be exercized in their use and interpretation. In any case general scales should be used only to supplement menopause-specific scales, which should always be the measure of first choice.

References

1. Ware I, Sherbourne CD. The Mos 36 item short-form survey (SF-36). *Med Care* 1992;30:473–83
2. Martin EA. *The Oxford Medical Dictionary.* Oxford: Oxford University Press, 2000:640
3. Utian WH. The International Menopause Society menopause-related terminology definitions. *Climacteric* 1999;2:284–6
4. Greene JG. The cross-sectional legacy: an introduction to longitudinal studies of the climacteric. *Maturitas* 1992;14:95–101
5. Holte A. Influences of natural menopause on health complaints: a prospective study of healthy Norwegian women. *Maturitas* 1992;14:127–41
6. Hunter M. The South East England longitudinal study of the climacteric and postmenopause. *Maturitas* 1992;14:117–26
7. Kaufert P, Gilbert P, Tate R. The Manitoba Project: a re-examination of the link between menopause and depression. *Maturitas* 1992;14:143–55
8. Avis N, Brambella D, McKinlay S, *et al.* A longitudinal analysis of the association between menopause and depression: results from the Massachusetts Women's Health Study. *Ann Epidemiol* 1994;4:214–20
9. Dennerstein L, Smith AMA, Morse C. Psychological well-being, mid-life and the menopause. *Maturitas* 1994;20:1–11
10. Collins A, Landgren BM. Reproductive health, use of oestrogen and experience of symptoms in perimenopausal women: a population-based study. *Maturitas* 1995;20:101–11
11. Woods NF, Mitchell ES. Patterns of depressed mood in mid-life women: observations from the Seattle Mid-life Women's Health Study. *Res Nurs Health* 1996;19:111–23
12. Peck D, Shapiro C. *Measuring Human Problems; A Practical Guide.* Chichester: Wiley, 1990
13. Kupperman HS, Wetchler BB, Blatt MH. Contemporary therapy of the menopausal syndrome. *J Am Med Assoc* 1959;171:1627–37
14. Alder E. The Blatt Kupperman Menopausal Index: a critique. *Maturitas* 1998;29:19–24
15. Beck AT, Ward CH, Mendelson M, *et al.* An inventory for measuring depression. *Arch Gen Psychiatry* 1961;4:561–74
16. Campbell S, Whitehead M. Oestrogen therapy and the menopausal syndrome. *Clin Obstet Gynaecol* 1977;4:31–47
17. Schneider M, Brotherton P, Hailes J. The effect of exogenous oestrogen on depression in menopausal women. *Med J Aust* 1977;2:162–3
18. Dernerstein L, Burrows GD, Hyman G, *et al.* Hormone therapy and affect. *Maturitas* 1979;1:247–59
19. Channon LD, Ballanger SE. Some aspects of sexuality and vaginal symptoms during the menopause and their relation to anxiety and depression. *Br J Med Psychol* 1986;59:173–80
20. Derman RJ, Dawood MY, Stone S. Quality of life during sequential hormone replacement therapy – a placebo controlled study. *Int J Fertil* 1995;40:73–8
21. Portin R, Polo-Kantola P, Polo O, *et al.* Serum oestrogen level, attention, memory and other cognitive functions in middle-aged women. *Climacteric* 1999;2:115–23
22. Khoo SK, Coglan M, Battistutta D, *et al.* Hormonal treatment and psychological function during menopause transition: an evaluation of conjugated oestrogens/cyclic medroxyprogesterone acetate. *Climacteric* 1998;1:55–62
23. Nagata C, Shimizu R, Takami R, *et al.* Hot flushes and other menopausal symptoms in relation to soy product intake in Japanese women. *Climacteric* 1999;2:6–12
24. Radloff LS. The CES–D scale: a self-report depression scale for research in the general population. *J Appl Psychol Meas* 1997;1:385–401
25. Ballanger CB. Psychiatric morbidity and the menopause: screening of general population sample. *Br Med J* 1975;3:344–6
26. Spearman C. General intelligence objectively determined and measured. *Am J Psychol* 1904;15:202–93
27. Eysenck HJ. *The Scientific Structure of Personality.* London: Keegan Paul, 1952
28. Cattell RB. *Personality and Motivation: Structure and Measurement.* London: Harrap, 1957
29. Eysenck HJ. The classification of depressive illness. *Br J Psychiatry* 1970;117:241–50
30. Hamilton M. The assessment of anxiety states by rating. *Br J Med Psychol* 1959;32:50–5
31. Lawley DN, Maxwell AE. *Factor Analysis as a Statistical Method.* London: Butterworth, 1963
32. Child D. *The Essentials of Factor Analysis.* London: Holt, Rinehart and Winston, 1976
33. Jaszman L. A plea for a uniform menopausal index. Fourth International Congress on the Menopause, Orlando, 1984; Abstract 14
34. Utian W. Menopause, sex hormones and quality of life. Sixth International Congress on the Menopause, Bangkok 1990; Abstract 160
35. Heinemann K, Assman A, Möhrer S, *et al.* Reliability of the Menopause Rating Scale. *Zentralbl Gynakol* 2002;124:157–9
36. Greene JG. A factor analytic study of climacteric symptoms. *Psychosom Res* 1976;20:425–30
37. Greene JG. *The Social and Psychological Origins of the Climacteric Syndrome.* Aldershot and Brookfield: Gower, 1984

38. Greene JG. *Guide to the Greene Climacteric Scale.* Glasgow: Glasgow University Press, 1991

39. Greene JG. Constructing a standard climacteric scale. *Maturitas* 1998;29:25–31

40. Hunter M, Battersby R, Whitehead M. Relationships between psychological symptoms, somatic complaints and menopausal status. *Maturitas* 1986;8:217–28

41. Hunter M. The Women's Health Questionnaire: a measure of mid-aged women's perceptions of their emotional and physical health. *Psychology and Health* 1992;7:45–54

42. Hunter M. The Women's Health Questionnaire (WHQ): development, standardization and application of a measure of mid-aged women's emotional and physical health. *Qual Life Res* 2001;9;733–8

43. Perz JM. Development of the Menopause Symptom Checklist. A factor analytic study of menopause associated symptoms. *Women and Health* 1997;25:53–69

44. Schneider H, Heinemann L, Rosemeier H-P, *et al.* The Menopause Rating Scale (MRS): reliability of scores of menopausal complaints. *Climacteric* 2000;3:59–64

45. Schneider H, Heinemann L, Rosemeier H-P, *et al.* The Menopause Rating Scale (MRS): comparison with Kupperman Index and quality-of-life scale SF-36. *Climacteric* 2000;3: 50–8

46. Utian WH, Janata JW, Kingsberg SA, *et al.* Determinants and quantification of quality of life after the menopause: the Utian Menopause Quality of Life score. In Aso T., ed. *The Menopause at the Millennium.* Carnforth: Parthenon Publishing, 2000:141–4

Contemporary evaluation of climacteric complaints: its impact on quality of life

4

H. P. G. Schneider and H. M. Behre

INTRODUCTION

The climacteric is a period of life encompassing those years in which a woman passes through a transition, from the reproductive stage of life to the menopausal years – a period marked by waning ovarian function. The point of time when cessation of menstruation occurs is referred to as menopause.

The Massachusetts Women's Health Study[1] provided data from 2570 women with a median age for the onset of menopause of 51.3 years. Only current smoking could be identified as a cause of earlier menopause, a shift of approximately 1.5 years. Those factors that were not found to affect the onset of menopause were oral contraception, socio-economic status and marital status. The age range of menopause is approximately 48–55. The perimenopausal transition, for most women, lasts for approximately four years.

Mothers and daughters tend to experience menopause at the same age, as suggested by clinical experience. However, appropriate longitudinal studies are missing, as is the case with the influence of ethnic differences. Undernourished women will experience an earlier menopause[2]. There is also no correlation between age of menarche and age of menopause[3].

Thinner women experience a slightly earlier menopause[4], obviously related to the contribution of body fat to estrogen production. Factors of little influence are race, income, geography, parity and height[1,4].

Most historical investigation indicates that the age of menopause has changed little since early Greek times[5]. An earlier menopause is associated with living at high altitudes and with cigarette smoking. Premature ovarian failure can occur in women who have previously undergone abdominal hysterectomy, presumably because ovarian vasculature has been compromised[6].

RECOGNITION OF THE IMPORTANCE OF HOW PATIENTS COPE WITH THE IMPACT OF CLIMACTERIC SYMPTOMS

The cessation of menses by most women is perceived as not influencing subsequent physical and mental health[1]. Women tend to express either positive or neutral feelings about menopause with the exceptions of those who experience surgical menopause[1]. By that token, the majority of women who feel healthy and happy do not seek contact with physicians. Medical intervention at this point of life should rather be regarded as an opportunity to provide and reinforce a program of preventive healthcare[7]. These issues of preventive healthcare for women include family planning, cessation of smoking, control of body weight and alcohol consumption, prevention of heart disease and osteoporosis, maintenance of mental well-being (including sexuality), cancer screening and treatment of neurological problems.

Leon Speroff[7] has phrased menopause as a wonderful signal occurring at the right time of life when preventive healthcare is especially critical. This positive attitude would require an understanding of the epidemiology of menopause, an understanding that is based on the recognition of this event as a normal stage in development. Development – a broader

Animal studies have suggested that estrogen inhibits the development of atherosclerosis independent of lipids. Estrogen and progesterone receptors have been identified in the endothelium and smooth muscle of human arterial vessels. Estrogens influence hemodynamics by increasing cardiac output and decreasing peripheral vascular resistance. They have been shown to increase cerebral blood flow and cognitive function. The relative risk of coronary heart disease was shown to be decreased in postmenopausal estrogen users. Estrogen has a favorable impact on serum and lipoprotein profiles. Prospective, randomized and controlled trials (Women's Health Initiative) are expected to present data on the real impact of primary and secondary cardiovascular prevention with sexual hormones.

Other long-standing metabolic consequences of the climacteric include osteoporosis and osteoporotic fractures, skin changes, weight gain and obesity and degenerative disease of the central nervous system (CNS). There is still much to be discovered and learned about the action of estrogen and other sex steroids on immunity, CNS function or musculo-skeletal disease, particularly at the cellular level. Specific forms of treatment with increased benefits and fewer risks are sought. But in particular, the knowledge of symptoms and their effect on the daily lives of women will assist the caregiver to provide competent care and provide women with long-standing professional assistance during the aging process. For that reason, it will be very helpful to provide objective information on individual disposition to symptoms of the climacteric and their impact on quality of life (QoL).

CONVENTIONAL VARIABLES SUPPLEMENTED WITH SELF-ASSESSMENT MEASURES FOR EVALUATION OF TREATMENT EFFECTS

In recent years, there has been a growing awareness among clinicians of the importance of learning more about how patients cope with the symptoms of their condition. Health-related quality of life is a subjective parameter commonly used to assess the views of the patients in terms of the physical, social and emotional aspects of living with their condition. Direct questioning is a simple and appropriate way of accruing information about how patients feel and function. The health-related QoL measures, whatever their theoretical basis, are generated from subjective responses and open to substantial methodological criticism and are often performed with less quantitative rigour[12]. Using standard questionnaires, however, does ensure that these psychometric properties are well documented. For routine application in clinical practice or in clinical trials, it is essential that the instruments employed are simple and comparatively short. To the doctors, paramedics and psychologists involved, a critical question has always been whether or not psychologic studies upset patients. The majority of patients or probands, however, welcome the opportunity to report how symptoms and their subsequent treatment affect daily life[13].

Psychometrically evaluated questionnaires allow uniform administration and unbiased quantification of data, as the response options are pre-determined and thus equal for all respondents[12]. A core set of questionnaires would allow the comparison of study results and patient populations. The growing awareness of an interest in the subjective aspects of QoL outcomes is evident by increasing numbers of publications in this area, with a growing emphasis on self-administered questionnaires. Unless conventional variables are supplemented with self-assessment measures, a limited picture of the impact of symptoms and the effect of treatment is obtained. Certain aspects may act together to introduce bias to interpretation. For example, interviewed individuals – particularly of older age – might have difficulty with reading or writing, or may be exposed to interviewers of varying experience. The expenses involved in gathering QoL data may also have an influence. Standardization, compatibility, eradication of possible bias and economy are therefore important variables of validity in any type of QoL assessment.

The application of health-related QoL instruments requires the same scrutiny and attention as the measurement of physiological outcomes. Random and representative samples of the population should be investigated in sufficient numbers and over prolonged periods of time. In terms of statistics QoL is, by definition, a multi-state attribute. The use of many measures in the multiple statistical tests reduces the statistical power of the analysis[14]. Health-related QoL certainly is a multi-dimensional concept; there is a continuing debate on whether or not the aggregation of several dimensions into a summary index is appropriate. A summary score may falsely suggest improvement in one vital area and conceal deterioration in another[14]. Indices, however, are practical and are a convenient method of information transfer.

HEALTH-RELATED QUALITY OF LIFE IN CLIMACTERIC WOMEN

Increasing age is accompanied by poorer health, as manifested by higher disease rates and increasing levels of frailty and disability. There is a tremendous amount of variation in the manner in which individuals age and respond to illness. Consequently, knowledge of a patient's baseline function in health is critical for accurate diagnosis and therapy. In the medical context, use of the concept of QoL is deliberately confined to health-related QoL[15]. The most important and universally accepted domains reflect physical, emotional and social functioning[16].

QoL assessments have many potential applications in clinical practice. If one tries to relate the broad aspects of menopausal symptoms to general well-being, and explore the extent to which the symptoms may influence a postmenopausal woman's QoL, clearly this asks for the potential of appropriate assessments. This would enable physicians and healthcare personnel to follow individual variation during the climacteric and also verify the effects of any kind of treatment.

Assessing the impact of a condition on QoL is particularly relevant in symptomatic con-

ditions such as the climacteric. The growing importance of all aspects of personal well-being and QoL can be summarized as a paradigmatic change in the definition of health:

(1) The World Health Organization definition, besides somatic aspects, also covers the psychologic and social components of health;

(2) Demographic variation with a growing population of elderly is associated with incremental chronic illness; it is appropriate to promote as a goal the status of healthy and independent elders who maintain physical and cognitive function as long as possible; and

(3) Rather than looking at classical therapeutic targets, such as reduction of symptoms or extension of life-time, optimal health strategies to incremental chronic illness should rather be defined as changing the slope or the rate at which illness develops; thus, clinical illness can be postponed, and if this is done for long enough, effectively be prevented.

In order to improve the individual's sense of controlling age-affected health, QoL assessment becomes more and more important. Monitoring variations in physical, emotional and social life parameters, as indicators of improvement of QoL and general well-being, is also important for the discussion of the cost-effectiveness of new therapeutic strategies targeted to reduce morbidity in the elderly.

The assessment of QoL and its aspects of methodology are described in Chapter 1. Of the various instruments developed for measuring QoL, two basic types of questionnaires exist: generic and disease- or treatment-specific. Although QoL may be defined in different ways, the contents of the different generic scales show many similarities, assessing the ability of patients to cope with their condition physically, emotionally and socially as well as their general performance at work and in daily life[17]. Among the more commonly used instruments are the Sickness Impact Profile[18], the Nottingham Health

Profile[19], Quality of Well-Being Scale[20], or the Short Form (SF)-36 Health Survey[21]. The generic measures cover the multi-dimensional aspects of QoL in a wide range of health problems. They might be less responsive to treatment-induced changes, and may be lengthy and time-consuming.

In contrast, the disease-specific measures are more likely to be responsive and make sense to both clinicians and patients. Their specific items relate to concepts and domains in patients' populations, diagnostic groups or diseases. One of the first, and still dominant, is the Women's Health Questionnaire (WHQ), a menopause-specific instrument[22]. The WHQ consists of 37 items including nine scales and it assesses, in addition to vasomotor symptoms, important areas such as other somatic symptoms, mood, sleep problems, cognitive difficulties and sexual functioning. Other test systems and questionnaires refer to psychiatric problems, pain scores, sleep disturbances, sexual dysfunction, mental and cognitive function.

DEVELOPMENT OF THE MENOPAUSE RATING SCALE

The first widely accepted attempt to measure the severity of menopausal complaints in women was the Kupperman Index[23,24]. The focus of this instrument primarily is on symptomatic relief, assessed on the basis of the physician's summary of the severity of climacteric complaints and assisted by the index rather than a woman's independent response. Our own attempt was to establish an instrument that can easily be filled in by patients. Therefore, we had a newly developed Menopause Rating Scale (MRS) specifically validated[25,26].

In 1996, a questionnaire was completed by a representative random sample of 689 German women aged 40–60 years in order to evaluate the newly established MRS. The MRS produces a total score of eleven specific menopausal symptoms, and scores on three independent dimensions: severity of somatic, psychologic and urogenital symptoms (Table 1). A follow-up investigation was organised in August–

October 1997 with a random sample of those women who already participated in 1996. The purpose was to characterize the stability of individual scores, and to identify possible reasons for variation of the scores over time. A total of 306 women completed our follow-up questionnaire. Additional aspects of - the questionnaire relate to menopausal transition, drug effects on menopausal complaints and a variation of new medical conditions with the aging process.

The changes of the MRS scores were stratified by the height of the initial score, estimated by mean and standard deviation; as a measure of the similarity of the scores both Pearson's correlation and Kendall's Tau-b were applied. Differences among the score level categories at entry regarding the mean increase or decrease, respectively, were tested by the Student's t-test. Unconditional regression analyses were performed adjusting for potential confounders in order to identify important factors that may have an impact on the increase or decline of MRS scores. SAS and STATA statistical packages were used.

Population-based standardization

The characteristics of our cohort of 306 women participating in a follow-up study are listed in Table 2. Almost all of the characteristics of our sample changed with time: the menopause status, most of the diseases reported, and the treatment of menopausal complaints. The mean age of the group grew from 49.6 (± 6.2) years at entry to 51.2 (± 6.2). At follow-up, 37% of the women were over 55 years old, 30% were pensioners and 73% were married or lived in stable partnership. A total of 48% still remained in the premenopausal phase of the climacteric transition while 52% experienced a postmenopausal state. In the years since the baseline survey, 14% of the sample contacted a physician due to menopausal symptoms. One-fifth of the participants estimated their health as less than satisfactory, and 21% reported a deterioration since the baseline survey. Hypertension, joint/muscle complaints and lower back pain were the most frequently reported health issues.

Table 1 Menopause Rating Scale

MENOPAUSE RATING SCALE (MRS)					
	Degree of severity				
Items	none no point	mild 1 point	moderate 2 points	severe 3 points	extremely severe 4 points
Hot flushes, sweating					
Anxiety					
Sleep disorders					
Irritability					
Depressive mood					
Heart symptoms					
Exhaustion					
Muscle & joint pain					
Sexual complaints					
Urinary symptoms					
Vaginal dryness					
Score $\Sigma \leq 44$ points					

Initially, about 38% of the participating women were on any remedy for their menopausal complaints; at follow-up 31% received treatment. Of those women seeking therapeutic assistance 28%, both peri- and postmenopausal, were using HRT at follow-up, 4% preferred phyto-hormones and 22% at some time were on psychotropic drugs.

Stability of test results

If one compares MRS scores at baseline and at follow-up investigation, some changes of the frequency of distribution are evident, as demonstrated in Table 3. The average deviation from the initial scores of the MRS was 2.0 (± 5.8). These changes were distributed among the scores in the somatic (0.8 ± 2.6), psychologic (0.5 ± 3) and urogenital (0.6 ± 1.9) dimensions. The frequency in the lowest

scoring category (0–4 points) declined over the observation period, while it grew in the higher categories. This tendency can also be observed for the three subscales. The majority of women remained in the category with no or mild complaints.

The mean decrease of the total score and the magnitude of score at the start of the observation are significantly associated. The higher the score at entry, the bigger the chance of a drop. There is no such relationship for increasing scores.

These results of our follow-up survey with the MRS demonstrate relatively stable individual scores unless intervening variables such as new diseases, treatments or other conditions occurred during the observational period. Obviously women without new medical conditions produce a higher level of stability of the MRS total score compared with those with

Table 2 Characteristics of a cohort of women participating in a follow-up investigation of the MRS

Variable	n	Category	Baseline n	Baseline %	Follow-up n	Follow-up %	Similarity* Value
Occupational status	306	Pensioner	39	13	40	13	0.55 (0.41; 0.69)
Marital status	306	Married or in stable partnership	229	75	222	73	0.88 (0.81; 0.94)
Menopausal status	306	Menses still regular	131	43	128	42	0.65 (0.57; 0.73)
		Menses irregular	28	9	19	6	
		No menses	147	48	159	52	
Contacts to health care	306	Due to menopausal complaints	53	17	42	14	0.34 (0.20; 0.48)
History of diseases†	246	Hypertension	61	20	70	23	0.59 (0.47; 0.70)
	230	Pain in the chest (Angina)	18	6	10	3	0.19 (−0.03; 0.41)
	232	Heart failure	17	6	17	6	0.25 (0.04; 0.46)
	233	Diabetes mellitus	11	4	11	4	0.62 (0.38; 0.87)
	257	Complaints of joints/ muscles	65	21	81	26	0.61 (0.51; 0.72)
	275	Lower back pain	150	49	168	55	0.43 (0.33; 0.53)
	233	Lung disease	16	5	26	9	0.46 (0.26; 0.65)
	238	Gastrointestinal diseases	27	9	27	9	0.35 (0.17; 0.53)
	233	Urinary tract conditions	11	4	17	6	0.41 (0.17; 0.65)
Drug treatment for menopausal complaints	306	Currently	68	22	95	31	0.56 (0.47; 0.66)
		Previously	14	5	22	7	
	130	Hormones (HRT)	56	18	87	28	0.45 (0.31; 0.58)
	130	Phytohormones	9	3	13	4	0.21 (−0.05; 0.48)
	306	Psychotropic drugs	69	23	68	22	0.37 (0.26; 0.48)

*measure of association among the two surveys: Kendall's tau-b values and 95% confidence interval;
†self-reported positive disease history

incident medical conditions. Multivariate analyses of the medical history including drug treatment, health status and contact with the healthcare system, besides age and a few social characteristics, give rise to a similar conclusion: a variation of scores and its direction are mainly influenced by health-related variables.

The majority of women demonstrated a stable level of complaints over the observational period. Differences in the MRS score at follow-up occurred with changes in health status. The MRS scores varied mainly with co-morbidity such as cardiac failure, chest pain, chronic gastrointestinal problems, rheumatoid or joint/muscle complaints and others. This variation over time is similar across various degrees of severity and menopausal complaints. Thus, a well-defined menopausal complaint self-rating scale serves the purpose of a less troublesome, practical and less time-consuming instrument to address the impact of any therapy on various aspects of QoL, and at the same time avoid interpersonal bias of patients and health personnel. Introducing

Table 3 MRS scores at baseline and follow-up investigation

a) Total score*
(mean difference baseline–follow-up: 2 ± 5.8)

Scoring points	Baseline		Follow-up	
	n	%	n	%
0–4	147	48.0	97	31.7
5–8	76	24.8	89	29.1
9–2	41	13.4	52	17.0
13–16	25	8.2	36	11.7
17+	17	5.6	32	10.5

b) Score of the somatic dimension*
(mean difference baseline–follow-up: 0.8 ± 2.6)

Scoring points	Baseline		Follow-up	
	n	%	n	%
0–4	235	76.8	197	64.4
5–8	56	18.3	85	27.8
9–12	13	4.2	20	6.5
13–16	2	0.7	4	1.3

c) Psychologic score*
(mean difference baseline–follow-up: 0.5 ± 3)

Scoring points	Baseline		Follow-up	
	n	%	n	%
0–4	247	80.7	233	76.1
5–8	49	16.0	52	17.0
9–12	7	2.3	18	5.9
13–16	3	1.0	3	1.0

d) Score of complaints in the urogenital tract*
(mean difference baseline–follow-up: 0.6 ± 1.9)

Scoring points	Baseline		Follow-up	
	n	%	n	%
0–4	298	97.4	282	92.2
5–8	7	2.3	23	7.5
9–12	1	0.3	1	0.3

*$p < 0.0001$, statistical agreement between follow-up and baseline according to K statistics

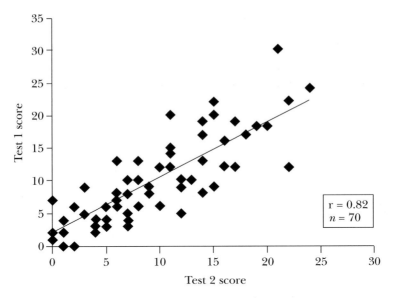

Figure 1 Test–retest reliability of the basic MRS. The test was answered twice with a time interval of about two weeks by 70 female volunteers aged 45–65 years. r, Pearson's correlation coefficient

the MRS into medical practice would result in improved co-operation and a higher degree of long-term compliance.

Linguistic and cultural translation and validation into English

We conducted a translation and cultural validation of the MRS scale, originally developed in German, into English for use in North America and the United Kingdom[27]. Following international methodological recommendations, the MRS scale was translated in a standardized way consisting of forward translation, quality control, backward translation and a pretest. Five experienced bilingual translators and reviewers were involved.

Many difficulties of compatibility between the cultural background of Germany, the UK and North America were identified and resolved by consensus. This resulted in one version for British and American English (Table 4). A pretest in volunteers demonstrated clarity and understandability across social classes, but also suggested minor changes in the instrument. A basic test–retest comparison of the MRS scale showed high

reliability with a correlation coefficient of over 0.8 for the total score (Figure 1).

Comparison with Kupperman Index

In their key publication on the revision of a menopausal index, Herbert Kupperman and his associates[24] argued that: "Nature has so endowed human beings that ovarian failure and incapacity for conception takes place at an age when the potential for both foetal abnormalities and complications in pregnancy increases, simply on the basis of age; why the ovary alone is singled out to become the 'Achilles heel' of the glands of internal secretion, is not understood. Beneficial as it may appear from the standpoint of eugenics and pure obstetrics, cessation of ovarian function does create certain disadvantages in many women."

Based on his contemporary resumé of menopausal physiology, Kupperman pointed to the fact that laboratory tests to detect hormonal insufficiency were too complicated and not precise enough, such that the clinician was dependent on symptoms of the climacteric to diagnose the condition of his patient. In other words, Kupperman was essentially bio-

Table 4 Schematic flow chart of the standardized translation process

Menopause Rating Scale (MRS)

Which of the following symptoms apply to you at this time?
Please mark the appropriate box for each symptom. For symptoms that do not apply, please mark 'none'.

	Symptoms:			
	none	*mild*	*moderate*	*severe*
Score:	0	1	2	3
Hot flushes, sweating (episodes of sweating)	☐	☐	☐	☐
Heart discomfort (unusual awareness of heart beat, heart skipping, heart racing, tightness)	☐	☐	☐	☐
Sleep problems (difficulty in falling asleep, difficulty in sleeping through, waking up early)	☐	☐	☐	☐
Depressive mood (feeling down, sad, on the verge of tears, lack of drive, mood swings)	☐	☐	☐	☐
Irritability (feeling nervous, inner tension, feeling aggressive)	☐	☐	☐	☐
Anxiety (inner restlessness, feeling panicky)	☐	☐	☐	☐
Physical and mental exhaustion (general decrease in performance, impaired memory, decrease in concentration, forgetfulness)	☐	☐	☐	☐
Sexual problems (change in sexual desire, in sexual activity and satisfaction)	☐	☐	☐	☐
Bladder problems (difficulty in urinating, increased need to urinate, bladder incontinence)	☐	☐	☐	☐
Dryness of vagina (sensation of dryness or burning in the vagina, difficulty with sexual intercourse)	☐	☐	☐	☐
Joint and muscular discomfort (pain in the joints, rheumatoid complaints)	☐	☐	☐	☐

THANK YOU VERY MUCH FOR YOUR COOPERATION

Table 5 Kupperman Index versus Menopause Rating Scale: item-to-item comparison

Kupperman Index	MRS
Vasomotor	Hot flushes, sweating
Paresthesia	Anxiety
Insomnia	Sleep disorders
Nervousness	Irritability
Melancholia	Drepressive mood
Vertigo	Heart symptoms
Weakness (fatigue)	Exhaustion
Arthralgia & myalgia	Muscle & joint pain
Headache	Sexual complaints
Palpitation	Urinary symptoms
Formication	Vaginal dryness

Six symptoms are roughly compatible, the other underlined five are not

assaying his patients. The principal handicap in determining the effectiveness of endocrine therapy in human beings was judged as being two-fold: one due to the pharmacological action of the drug itself and the other to the psychological influence of drug administration. For that matter, the most prominent symptoms of the climacteric were used in formulating a numerical conversion index designated as the menopausal index.

After more than 40 years of progress in endocrine research, and with its current and widespread immunoassay-based diagnostics and more subtle insight into psycho-neuroendocrine control of human behavior and well-being, the practicing physician still depends on a reliable and easy-to-manage evaluation of the climacteric syndrome.

Kupperman's proposals for a quantitative evaluation of menopausal symptoms enabled generations of physicians to adequately evaluate symptomatology and the success of various treatments. Later on during the 1970s, the first placebo-controlled and randomized cross-over studies were done to further specify menopausal symptoms[28,29]. We felt it necessary to develop a menopause-specific QoL instrument according to new standards, such as self-administration, in a representative population-based sample. This was the reason for developing and standardizing a new MRS. For its further evaluation, we applied in

parallel the most widely used Kupperman Index. This Kupperman Index lists 11 menopausal symptoms in their sequence of importance. Table 5 shows how this matches with the MRS.

The Kupperman Index includes a severity rating of the individual symptoms by means of a weighting factor corresponding to their importance. The symptom 'vasomotor' – covering hot flushes, perspiration and night sweats – is given a weighting factor of four, whereas the symptoms of paresthesia, insomnia and nervousness have a weighting factor of two. The remaining symptoms, namely melancholia, vertigo, weakness, arthralgia and myalgia, headaches, palpitation and formication are giving a weight of only one. Furthermore, the Kupperman Index recognizes four grades of severity for each symptom that act as multiplication factors for the index. The complaints are rated by the physician in contrast to the MRS which is directly administered to women. The final scores of the Kupperman Index are more difficult to calculate, particularly as the MRS weights any symptom as equal. For comparison between the two scales, the Kupperman Index has been adopted[26].

A total of six complaints are roughly identical between the Kupperman Index and the MRS score, and five non-compatible symptom complexes exist in each scale. In practice, the Kupperman Index has the following categories for degrees of severity of menopausal symptoms: 35 points or more refers to severe symptoms; 20–34 points refers to moderate symptoms; and 15–19 points refers to mild symptoms.

Kupperman was considering a therapeutic regimen as efficacious if it would reduce the index to a level of 15 or less. A further differentiation of scores below 15 is originally not defined, but we separated two additional categories: 1–14 points referring to minor symptoms and no points referring to no complaints.

The results of both scales were cross-calculated. The distribution of each scale was divided into quartiles, because the usual categories (mild, moderate or severe complaints) do not necessarily have identical meaning across the instruments. The results of both instruments were closely associated. However, there seems to be a difference in the association among the quartiles. The highest quartile depicts a higher congruence in scoring (80%), whereas the middle and lower quartiles show a greater deviation. More women were classified in the lowest quartile with the MRS (31.7%) than with the Kupperman Index (25.8%). While 67% of the women in the lowest quartile of MRS were also classified in this quartile by the Kupperman Index, 29.9% and 3% were found in the second and third quartile respectively of the Kupperman scale. The lowest agreement with Kupperman's Index was observed in the second quartile of MRS results[26].

More of a difference becomes apparent if one considers the categories mild, moderate and severe complaints as identical in both instruments and then tries to compare the original data. The categories 'mild' and 'severe' menopausal symptoms collected only 38% of the women according to the original evaluation scheme of the Kupperman Index. In other words, 62% of the participants are not sufficiently defined by the original categories of the Kupperman Index with their index ranging from 0–14 points. On the other hand, if one aggregates the original categories 'no' to 'mild' symptoms in both scales, 31% and 77%

of the sample are classified to MRS and Kupperman, respectively. These weighting differences need to be considered when looking at the original categories of severity of menopausal symptoms obtained with both instruments[26].

Altogether, the scoring results of both MRS and Kupperman Index are measuring the same condition. However, when the original degrees of severity of both scales are analyzed, caution is required: the terms 'mild', 'moderate' and 'severe' menopausal complaints reflect different contents. The MRS scale defines the cut-off points between degrees of severity in accordance with a population survey. The Kupperman Index utilizes patients as a reference, and consequently classifies many more women in a population sample in the 'no/minor' category compared to the MRS. Thus, both scales are differently spread and not directly compatible.

If one tries to adopt the differences in the denominators of both the MRS and the Kupperman Index, and introduces quartiles to both scales, we are still left with the following additional differences among the two scales:

(1) Although both indices apparently measure an identical biological condition, the MRS seems to be more economic than the Kupperman Index in three ways: (a) the scoring is done by women themselves. The physician is not confronted with additional efforts of documentation; (b) the calculation of the total index of MRS is relatively simple, as there is no rating and multiplication of factors involved; and (c) the index categories of MRS differentiate more appropriately in the higher-degree symptoms compared with the Kupperman Index. There is a population-adopted spread in the categories of the MRS.

(2) In a non-clinical representative population survey, a large number of women are listed at symptom levels which are not defined by the classified Kupperman Index.

(3) The psychometric quality of the MRS in many ways is adequately standardized when compared to the Kupperman Index.

Relation with quality of life assessment by SF-36

In order to adequately assess well-being in menopausal women, a defined QoL measure has to be considered. During their fifth decade of life, women will experience a noticeable general decrease in QoL. This phenomenon is not only restricted to menopausal transition. The pertinent question, however, is how much of the generic QoL is reflected in the MRS? One of the most widely accepted measurement systems is the SF-36 Health Survey which depicts generic health concepts relevant across age, disease and treatment groups[21]. It provides a comprehensive, psychometrically sound and efficient way to measure health from the patient's point of view by scoring standardized responses to standardized questions.

Eight multi-item scales of the SF-36 have been analyzed. We compared the somatic sum-score of SF-36 with the score of the somatic dimension of MRS, subdivided into quartiles (Table 6a). The agreement between both scales is highest in the first and last quartile of the MRS distribution; the direction of both scales is opposite (MRS and SF-36 measuring increase in pathology and health, respectively). Generally, the higher the score in the somatic dimensions of the MRS, the lower the QoL according to the somatic sum-score of the SF-36.

A similar relation was found for the psychological sum-scores of both scales (Table 6b). The analysis has also been stratified according to age. No remarkable difference was seen.

In order to depict the relation of menopausal complaints with QoL more clearly, we looked at the complete eight multi-item scales of the SF-36 in relation to the four quartiles of the MRS degrees of severity (Figure 2). The mean values of most of the dimensions of SF-36 differ somewhat among groups of women with different degrees of menopausal complaints (quartiles of MRS). The loss of QoL is maximal in women with severe menopausal symptoms (upper quartile of

Table 6 Association of SF-36 and MRS sum-scores: a, somatic sum-score of MRS and SF-36; b, psychologic sum-score of MRS and SF-36

a) Somatic sum-scores of MRS and SF-36

SF-36 Quartiles	MRS								Total
	n	%	n	%	n	%	n	%	
1.	7	9.1	10	15.4	30	35.3	24	53.3	71
2.	7	9.1	24	36.9	32	37.7	12	26.7	75
3.	29	37.7	19	29.2	17	20	7	15.6	72
4.	34	44.2	12	18.5	6	7.1	2	4.4	54
Total	77	100	65	100	85	100	45	100	272

b) Psychologic sum-scores of MRS and SF-36

SF-36 Quartiles	MRS								Total
	n	%	n	%	n	%	n	%	
1.	5	4.9	3	7.3	20	29.9	42	68.9	70
2.	21	20.4	14	34.2	21	31.3	15	24.6	71
3.	45	43.7	12	29.3	16	23.4	4	6.6	77
4.	32	31.1	12	29.3	10	14.9	0	0	54
Total	103	100	41	100	67	100	61	100	272

34 women with missing answers in the SF-36 were excluded (= value 0); both scales were subdivided into quartiles

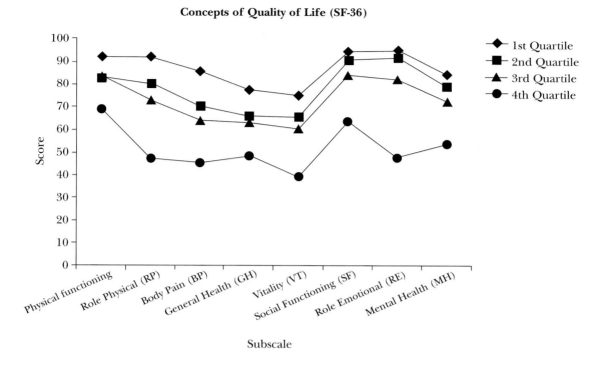

Figure 2 Complete SF-36 multi-item scores with MRS in relation to the four quartiles of MRS degrees of severity

MRS), less pronounced in those with no or mild symptoms (lower quartile), and not very different in the two middle quartiles of severity of menopausal complaints (MRS). These differences in the subscales of the SF-36 are most evident in role functioning – physical (RP), bodily pain (BP), vitality (VT) and role functional – emotional (RE), and much less in the remainder of the scales. Thus, the degree of severity of menopausal symptoms, measured with the MRS, clearly reflects the profile of the QoL dimensions of SF-36.

SUMMARY AND CONCLUSION

Originally, a group of experts of the German-speaking menopause societies reviewed the modern experience with symptoms specifically related to menopause and arrived at a list of eleven such items[25]. Practical experience with this newly established 'Menopause Rating Scale' (MRS) was published elsewhere[30–32]. The

definition of the MRS somatic subscale encompasses somatic complaints such as hot flushes, vasomotor symptoms, insomnia and musculo-skeletal disorders. The psychologic dimension consists of complaints like depression, irritability, anxiety and mental exhaustion. Depression is the collective term that relates to 'melancholia' with Kupperman. It is a reactive process and often termed 'depressive mood' or 'moodiness'. Mental exhaustion is related to 'lack of energy' or 'tiredness', or terms such as 'weakness' and 'fatigue'. It also implies 'poor concentration' and 'forgetfulness'. The dimension of general symptoms was defined as sexual dysfunction, urological complaints and vaginal atrophy. Sexual function includes a reduction in sexual desire and reduced sexual activity and/or satisfaction. Urological complaints imply 'urgency', 'loss of urine' or 'incontinence'. Finally, vaginal atrophy is coincident with 'vaginal dryness' and 'dyspareunia'. In other words, there are similarities and clear differences with regard to the Kupperman Index.

A world-wide group of the Health Foundation including very well-known authors such as van Keep[33] and Jaszmann[34] performed careful epidemiological studies and arrived at the conclusion that, apart from hot flushes and genital atrophy, all other symptoms named by Kupperman might be non-specific. Somewhat later, Utian's group[28] made similar statements like the Dutch investigators, but this time based on biochemical hormone measurements such as plasma estradiol and gonadotropin assays. Based on the intervention of these study groups, again the symptoms of hot flushes and genital atrophy for years were considered as true menopausal symptoms. Other signs and symptoms were looked at as being merely "psychogenic consequences of the menopause". Campbell[29] categorized these other symptoms in terms of a 'domino effect'.

The MRS proves to be more economic than the Kupperman Index. It measures specific menopausal symptoms, it categorizes the degree of symptoms more appropriately within a representative population and its psychometric quality is in many ways more elaborated.

Our analyses also demonstrate the striking dependence of the MRS classification of menopausal symptoms on the QoL. The SF-36 profile is distinctly different among the four quartiles of the total MRS score. For both the somatic and psychologic sum-scores, significant positive associations were found between the MRS and SF-36 scores. For that matter, the MRS can be utilised as an age- and condition-specific measure of QoL. Women with an insufficient QoL might well sense their menopausal symptoms more profoundly than women with a high QoL. In other words, one could speculate whether or not a good QoL may be protective against the clinical manifestation of menopausal symptoms.

In general, the MRS has proven to be an extremely valuable modern tool for assessing menopausal complaints. Its psychometric and practical evaluation has been demonstrated. Linguistic validation procedures have allowed the MRS to assume its optimal applicability in a broader European and American context; longitudinal studies are under way. A larger investigation of a representative population in Berlin has also documented the practical applicability of the MRS[35]. A study of more than 4000 women in a phase-IV clinical trial with two different HRT protocols of post-marketing surveillance has recently been reported[32]. This intricately defined menopausal complaint rating scale may serve as a less troublesome, less time-consuming and more practical instrument to assess the impact of treatment on various aspects of quality of life and at the same time avoid wide-range batteries of questionnaires.

References

1. McKinlay SM, Brambilla DJ, Posner JG. The normal menopause transition. *Maturitas* 1992; 14:103–15
2. Matthews KA, Wing RR, Kuller LH, *et al.* Influences of natural menopause on psychological characteristics and symptoms of middle-aged healthy women. *J Consult Clin Psychol* 1990;58:345–51
3. Treloar AE. Menarche, menopause and intervening fecundability. *Hum Biol* 1974;46:89–107
4. MacMahon B, Worcester J. Age at menopause U.S. 1960–62. *Vital Health Stat* 1966;11:1–20
5. Amundsen DW, Diers CJ. The age of menopause in medieval Europe. *Hum Biol* 1973;45: 605–12
6. Siddle N, Sarrel P, Whitehead M. The effect of hysterectomy on the age at ovarian failure: identification of a subgroup of women with premature loss of ovarian function and literature review. *Fertil Steril* 1987;47:94–100
7. Speroff L. A signal for the future. In Lobo R, ed. *Treatment of the Postmenopausal Woman.* New York: Raven Press, 1994:1–8
8. Fries JF. Aging, illness, and health policy: implications of the compression of morbidity. *Perspect Biol Med* 1988;31:407–28

9. Fries JF. Aging, natural death and the compression of morbidity. *N Engl J Med* 1980;303: 130–5

10. Fries JF, Green LW, Levine S. Health promotion and the compression of morbidity. *Lancet* 1989; 1:481–3

11. Anda RF, Waller MN, Wooten KG, *et al.* Behavioral risk factor surveillance, 1988. CDC Surveillance Summaries. MMWR 1991:39;1–22

12. Wiklund I. Methods of assessing the impact of climacteric complaints on quality of life. *Maturitas* 1998;29:41–50

13. Fallowfield L, Baum M, Maguire GP. Do psychological studies upset patients? *J R Soc Med* 1987;80:59

14. Fletcher AE, Gore S, Jones D, *et al.* Quality of life measures in health care. II: Design, analysis and interpretation. *Br Med J* 1992;305:1145–8

15. Guyatt G, Veldhuyzen Van Zanten S, Feeny D, *et al.* Measuring quality of life in clinical trials: a taxonomy and review. *Can Med Assoc J* 1989;140: 1441–8

16. Spitzer WO. State of science 1986: quality of life and functional status as target variables for research. *J Chron Dis* 1987;40:465–71

17. Fitzpatrick R, Fletcher A, Gose S, *et al.* Quality of life measures in health care: I. Applications and issues in assessment. *Br Med J* 1992;305: 1074–7

18. Bergner M. Development, use and testing of the Sickness Impact Profile. In Walker S, Rosser M, eds. *Quality of Life Assessment: Key Issues in the 1990s*. Dordrecht: Kluwer Academic Press, 1993:201–9

19. Hunt SM, McKenna SP, McEwen J, *et al.* The Nottingham Health Profile: Subjective health and medical consultations. *Soc Sci Med* 1981; 15A:221–9

20. Kaplan RM, Anderson JP, Ganiats T. The Quality of Wellbeing Scale: rationale for a single quality of life index. In Walker S, Rosser M, eds. *Quality of Life Assessment: Key Issues in the 1990s*. Dordrecht: Kluwer Academic Press, 1995:65

21. McHorney CA, Ware JE, Raczek AE. The MOS 36-item Short-Form health status survey (SF-36): II. Psychometric and clinical tests of validity in measuring physical and mental health constructs. *Med Care* 1993;31:247–63

22. Hunter M. The Women's Health Questionnaire (WHQ): a measure of mid-aged women's perceptions of their emotional and physical health. *Psychology and Health* 1992;7:45–54

23. Kupperman HS, Blatt MHG, Wiesbaden H, *et al.* Comparative clinical evaluation of estrogen preparations by the menopausal and amenorrhoeal indices. *J Clin Endocrinol* 1953;13: 688–703

24. Kupperman HS, Wetchler BB, Blatt MHG. Contemporary therapy of the menopausal syndrome. *J Am Med Assoc* 1959;171:1627–37

25. Schneider HPG, Heinemann LAJ, Rosemeier HP, *et al.* The Menopause Rating Scale (MRS): reliability of scores of menopausal complaints. *Climacteric* 2000;3:59–64

26. Schneider HPG, Heinemann LAJ, Rosemeier HP, *et al.* The Menopause Rating Scale (MRS): comparison with Kupperman index and quality-of-life scale SF-36. *Climacteric* 2000;3: 50–8

27. Utian WH. Definitive Symptome der Postmenopause – unter Verwendung des vaginalen Parabasalzellindexes. In *Oestrogene in der Postmenopause*. Möglichkeiten der Endokrinologie. Bâle: Karger, 1975:79–100

29. Heinemann K, Assman A, Möhner S, *et al.* Reliability of the Menopause Rating Scale. *Zentralbl Gynakol* 2002;124:157–9

29. Campbell S. Double blind psychometric studies on the effects of natural estrogens on postmenopausal women. In Campbell S, ed. *The Management of the Menopause & Post-Menopausal Years*. Lancaster: MTP Press Limited, 1976: 149–58

30. Hauser GA, Huber IC, Keller PJ, *et al.* Evaluation der klimakterischen Beschwerden (Menopause Rating Scale [MRS]). *Zentralbl Gynakol* 1994;116:16–23

31. Schneider HPG, Doeren M. Traits for long-term acceptance of hormone replacement therapy – results of a representative German survey. *Eur Menopause J* 1996;3:94–8

32. Schneider HPG, Rosemeier HP, Schnitker J, *et al.* Application and factor analysis of the menopause rating scale [MRS] in a post-marketing surveillance study of Climen®. *Maturitas* 2000;37:113–24

33. Van Keep PA, Kellerhals JM. The ageing woman. In van Keep PA, Lauritzen C, eds. *Ageing and Estrogens. Front Hormone Research*. Bâle: Karger, 1973:160–73

34. Jaszmann L. Epidemiology of climacteric and post-climacteric complaints. In van Keep PA, Lauritzen C, eds. *Ageing and Estrogens. Front Hormone Research*. Bâle: Karger, 1973:22–34

35. Rosemeier HP, Schultz-Zehden B. Psychologische Aspekte des Klimakteriums. In Fischl IH, Huber JC, eds. *Menopause*. Vienna: Krause & Pachernegg, 1995:3–11

Measurement of quality of life specific for aging males

5

L. A. J. Heinemann, F. Saad and P. Pöllänen

INTRODUCTION

Like women, men experience an age-related decline of physical and mental capacity. Symptoms such as impaired memory, lack of concentration, nervousness, depression, insomnia, periodic sweating or hot flushes, bone and joint complaints and reduction of muscle mass occur.

In women, menopausal or climacteric symptoms are widely accepted by the term 'menopause' and are being treated. But complaints in aging males have rarely – in the past – been put into the perspective of hormonal involution (although Werner[1] reported the similarity of male complaints to those of women in this age span as early as in the 1940s). Arguments for and against the male climacteric, as well as its compatibility with the female situation, have been discussed ever since[2–4]. However, the goal would be to establish treatment schemes to improve body composition and increase muscle strength, and by this and other favorable effects to increase quality of life (QoL) in general for aging males. This requires discussion of the indication of hormonal replacement therapy, and diagnostic instruments to reliably measure changes of QoL related to potential treatment options.

How should one assess QoL in aging men in a standardized way? (i.e. comparable to the menopausal scales available for women in the same age span.) This requires several steps:

(1) Identification of complaints/symptoms of aging males, i.e. selection of all items relevant to QoL in this age span;

(2) Putting relevant items together in a raw instrument/questionnaire;

(3) Analysing dimensions of the raw instrument to distinguish items relevant to age-related QoL from those due to frequent diseases/conditions in this age span;

(4) Determination of reference values for a given population;

(5) Cross-cultural validation for other languages/cultures: standardized translation following international rules and determination of reference values; and

(6) Validation of the scale, which involves:

- Assessment of test–retest reliability of the instrument

- External validity against other QoL instruments specific for this age span

- External validity against other generic QoL instruments

- Construct validation: comparison with clinical entities or hormone values, changes after hormone replacement or other therapeutic measures directed at improving aging males' symptoms.

The problem with the identification of specific complaints for aging males is that very little has actually been investigated so far. Men are not expected to actively complain and they do not usually report symptoms unless explicitly asked about them. An additional question is: where is empirical evidence that males and females really differ concerning symptoms during aging?

EVOLUTION OF COMPLAINTS WITH AGING – A GENDER-SPECIFIC PHENOMENON?

Scope of comparisons

Based on many health interview and examination surveys performed in Germany – surveys that included questions regarding symptoms that are an integral part of 'menopause scales' such as the Kupperman Index[5], Menopause Rating Scale (MRS)[6] and 'Aging Males' Symptoms' Rating Scale (AMS)[7] – we analyzed sex-specific differences in the frequency of symptom prevalence. Obviously, it is not easy to distinguish between signs and symptoms of aging, so-called 'climacteric symptoms' and symptoms of diseases/conditions. Thus, the question was very general: to what extent does the prevalence of complaints in men differ from those in women in the course of aging, particularly in the age span when women experience their menopausal transition? In other words, are the complaints associated with the 'climacteric syndrome' specific only for women? And to what extent could they be found in males as well?

Methods used

The methods used were published elsewhere[8]. In brief, six population-based surveys were included in a pooled analysis where the original databases were accessible, even though most of these data were not published. The six databases were screened for relevant symptoms in males and females, respectively. However, we could not find all the symptom groups we were interested in for comparison. We counted the presence of each of the symptoms across all databases and the number of persons questioned about these symptoms. The sample size varied, because not all databases contained information about all symptoms, and one of the large databases consisted of several sub-databases all of which contained some relevant information.

The symptoms encountered in the databases reflect only the currently perceived situation of the persons, without making comparisons to other persons of the same age, or impairment with respect to the situation ten years ago or any other standard. This means, though, that the same symptom might be differently understood at the age of 30 or 60 and different in males or females (for example, 'heavy sweating'). This sort of shortcoming was unavoidable with a pooled database study aiming at hypothesis generation only. Altogether, information from 8598 males and 8810 females was available for pooled analysis.

Age- and sex-specific symptoms

The overall result from our analysis of population surveys is: there is a very similar age-dependent development of complaints for both sexes. Somatic, psychological and urogenital symptoms were found in all age groups, but with somewhat different frequency. To avoid mild symptoms diluting the expected increase of prevalence with age, we only looked at complaints that were perceived as subjectively important (at least moderate or severe). Table 1 shows the frequencies of such marked symptoms across age and sex groups. The proportion of marked symptoms is astonishingly similar in males and females over 50 years of age. Only the symptoms 'intolerance of cold and heat', 'complaints in joints and muscles' and 'depressive mood' seem to be more prevalent in women across all age groups.

Obviously, the perception of symptoms changes with age and might differ across gender. The same question might well be understood differently by respondents, if the question is not phrased specifically enough. This is an obvious problem in database studies, and could be a reason for the unexpectedly high prevalence of symptoms such as reduced well-being, reduced physical strength and complaints in joints and muscles in age groups under 40.

The symptom of 'sweating/eruption of

Table 1 Relative frequency of complaints observed[8] in population surveys by age group and gender: percentage of persons with important or severe symptoms. (Numbers vary because information about severity of complaints was not available in all databases.)

Complaints	Age group	Males		Females	
		n	Percent	n	Percent
Reduced well-being	< 30	1022	4	1127	6
	30–39	2123	6	2276	7
	40–49	2467	8	2143	12
	50–59	2386	16	2224	15
	60+	1311	21	1217	20
Somatic symptoms					
Exhaustion, decreased energy	< 30	466	6	501	18
	30–39	908	6	979	16
	40–49	1194	10	961	18
	50–59	1227	19	1139	25
	60+	896	22	768	24
Weakness, reduced muscle strength	< 30	466	20	1003	25
	30–39	909	21	1958	24
	40–49	1197	17	1590	25
	50–59	1229	26	1760	31
	60+	902	23	1316	27
Complaints in joints or muscles	< 30	466	39	502	54
	30–39	909	49	980	53
	40–49	1200	44	794	62
	50–59	1229	52	880	65
	60+	897	49	661	63
Heavy sweating, eruption of sweat	< 30	466	34	500	22
	30–39	907	35	981	23
	40–49	1197	25	965	30
	50–59	1226	24	1148	52
	60+	896	21	779	39
Intolerance to cold or heat	< 30	932	13	1001	21
	30–39	1815	16	1956	23
	40–49	2017	16	1591	26
	50–59	2124	21	1760	35
	60+	1449	20	1322	34
Dizziness, drowsiness, imbalance	< 30	466	4	502	20
	30–39	909	6	981	21
	40–49	1198	7	796	23
	50–59	1229	14	881	24
	60+	899	14	659	28
Sleeping disturbances	< 30	577	9	603	9
	30–39	1167	10	1216	14
	40–49	1468	15	1256	25
	50–59	1625	21	1593	41
	60+	1080	21	930	41

Continued

Table 1 Continued

		Males		Females	
Complaints	Age group	n	Percent	n	Percent
Psychological symptoms					
Feeling to have passed your peak	< 30	227	1	272	2
	30–39	288	1	320	4
	40–49	602	5	233	3
	50–59	603	10	255	7
	60+	561	17	197	6
Totally discouraged, arrived at dead point	< 30	227	0.4	272	0.4
	30–39	288	–	321	0.6
	40–49	600	2	233	1
	50–59	604	3	255	0.8
	60+	560	3	197	2
Problems with concentration	< 30	122	20	118	21
	30–39	317	25	263	24
	40–49	288	27	242	26
	50–59	259	33	215	27
	60+	93	34	84	31
Depressive mood, sad, tearful	< 30	–	–	–	–
	30–39	–	–	–	–
	40–49	381	7	169	28
	50–59	332	10	262	32
	60+	353	9	112	38
Urogenital symptoms					
Decrease in libido or sexual activity	< 30	–	–	–	–
	30–39	–	–	–	–
	40–49	373	5	161	16
	50-59	317	10	260	31
	60+	329	25	111	24
Decrease in potency	< 30	–	–	–	–
	30–39	–	–	–	–
	40–49	376	3	–	–
	50–59	324	13	–	–
	60+	342	31	–	–
Uro-vaginal problems	< 30	–	–	–	–
	30–39	–	–	–	–
	40–49	–	–	330	10
	50–59	–	–	518	23
	60+	–	–	220	23
Decrease in morning erections	< 30	–	–	–	–
	30–39	–	–	–	–
	40–49	364	4	–	–
	50–59	308	15	–	–
	60+	313	28	–	–

sweat' seems to be a good example of a communication problem: males and females understood the question differently. For women, there was an increasing prevalence with age, but the opposite was observed in men. Different reasons for sweating (such as physical exercise compared with unexpected hot flushes without obvious reason) might be one explanation. However, there was not sufficient information to differentiate in this regard. Additionally, women may have learned to expect and to perceive sweating in certain age groups more easily than men. How certain can one be that the answer to one question reflects the same content across age and sex groups? More research with methods of social science and psychology is required here.

Conclusion

Despite all the limitations inherent in a pooled study like this, it can be hypothesized that: (1) the symptomatology of women and men over the age of 50 is fairly similar; and (2) complaints that are usually associated with the menopausal transition in women can be found to a certain degree at younger ages and in aging males – they do not appear suddenly, but develop slowly. Possibly, it is too simple to assume that menopausal complaints in women can be explained just because women of a certain age are estrogen deficient – and very few males have a similarly clear testosterone deficiency. At least, symptoms of well-acknowledged menopausal scales were also found in males at the same age and in women young enough to reject hormonal deficiency as a good explanation. Thus, symptoms may reflect a complex picture of hormonal and non-hormonal aspects of aging itself. This, however, is no reason to exclude a beneficial effect of hormone treatment.

The development of symptoms during aging needs to be confirmed by other specifically designed research, preferably longitudinal studies, but certainly studies designed to test such hypotheses. On the other hand, we are tempted to believe that the findings may not be explained only by any methodological weaknesses of this study approach – specifically designed research will show if this opinion can be substantiated or not.

Although single symptoms are non-specific, it seems to be clear – at least for women – that if several complaints appear as a cluster, it becomes part of the age-specific syndrome. This is the basis of many scales measuring menopausal symptoms in women. Based on these scales it was repeatedly reported that menopausal women exhibit a typical cluster of complaints with three dimensions: somato-vegetative, psychological and urogenital symptoms, which are used for assessing the severity of menopausal complaints[5,6]. Recently, a similar scale was standardized for aging males and the analysis showed the same cluster of symptoms[7]. Similar clusters of symptoms across gender can be used as another argument to support the hypothesis that the 'climacteric syndrome' – or better, aging – is similar in women and men, irrespective of the different underlying hormonal background.

THE AGING MALES' SYMPTOMS RATING SCALE: QUALITY OF LIFE IN AGING MALES

Development of the scale: aims

A new symptom inventory was developed based on a short check list of complaints suggested by Vermeulen (unpublished and not formally standardized), and additional symptoms that we observed at different frequencies in males over 55 compared to under 40 years of age in population surveys (Figure 1). In a pre-phase, the modified and more comprehensive Vermeulen checklist was applied to patients to see whether they understood the meaning and wording, initially by interviewers, in an advanced stage as a self-administered form. We received feedback and changed the wording of the questions as long as we had reason to assume that the content remained unclear (despite examples in parentheses). A point was reached when the checklist converted from a 'physician's view' to a 'patient's' or 'respondent's view'. This led to a draft checklist of complaints that could be completed by patients without major problems in understanding.

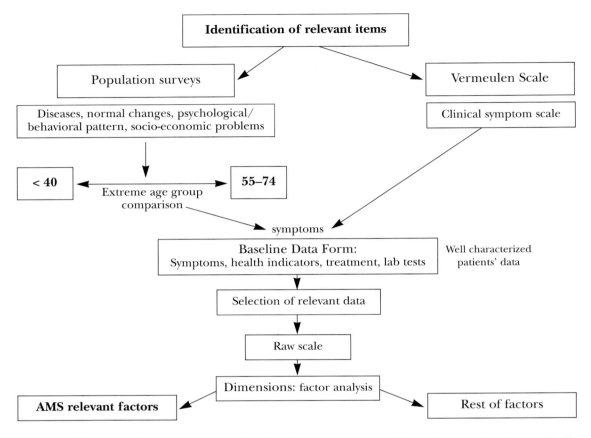

Figure 1 Schematic flow chart showing the identification of potential items for a QoL scale specifically related to aging males. The two sources (an existing symptom scale and an extreme group comparison) lead over several steps to items relevant for aging males

The objective of this first phase of the project was to specifically develop and test a scale that measures the symptoms (or quality of life, QoL) associated with aging in men (40–70 years), as experienced in the daily practice of health care. The AMS is easy to apply to patients and other lay persons. The intention was not to develop a standardized questionnaire for males suffering from androgen deficiency – as measured by testosterone levels in peripheral blood – i.e. not to develop a screening instrument for this specific group of males.

Sample to describe the dimensions of the scale

To achieve our goal, we decided to take a sample of medically well-characterized aging males in the first instance, i.e. to use GP practices as a sampling scheme rather than a random population sample. One hundred and sixteen thoroughly medically examined male patients aged over 40 years, and without serious acute or chronic disease or known hormonal problems, were recruited to gather information about aging males' symptoms and background parameters. Patients with minor diseases or early stages of medical conditions were included, but banal infections were preferred.

As a first task, all patients completed our draft symptoms inventory of 21 suspected aging males' symptoms. In addition to these specific symptoms, we tried to characterize the group regarding health care utilization, attitudes towards a healthy lifestyle/disease

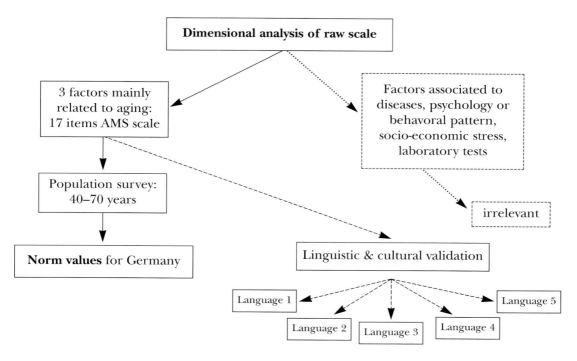

Figure 2 The process of determining dimensions of an aging-male-specific scale and further steps towards an applicable QoL instrument

prevention, disease history, use of certain drugs and some socio-economic characteristics, which might partly explain the so-called specific symptoms. Almost 200 parameters were recorded to distinguish between aging, diseases, psychosocial and other conditions. A description of the sample was published elsewhere[7].

Dimensions of aging males' symptoms

To put the various complaints or symptoms into perspective with aging, health problems or stressful situations the patient is exposed to, we analyzed the whole dataset with statistical methods that allow meaningful clustering of parameters/symptoms. To get characteristic profiles of symptoms for males aged 45–69, we applied factor analysis (principal component analysis with varimax rotation). Symptoms or complexes of inter-correlating symptoms formed 'dimensions' – it was intended to aggregate all relevant symptoms into a few dimensions of symptoms. We found a solution

with the dimensions[7] 'psychological', 'somato-vegetative' and 'sexual symptoms', which form clusters. These three factors account for 51.6% of the total variance of the raw AMS scale (21 items); two other factors were found to be related to diseases or conditions (additionally accounting for another 11% of the total variance) but are not further discussed here. Figure 2 depicts the process schematically.

Factor 1: psychological symptoms

This factor aggregates symptoms or complaints of a psychological nature in aging males. The five symptoms with the highest factor weights were discouragement, depression, irritability, anxiety and nervousness.

Factor 2: somato-vegetative symptoms

This dimension describes a complex of somatic and vegetative symptoms. The seven most important symptoms of this complex are painful symptoms in muscles or joints, sweating ('hot flushes'), increased need for sleep and sleep disturbances, impaired general well-being, decrease in muscular strength and decreased energy (exhaustion).

Factor 3: sexual complaints

This dimension basically consists of five symptoms only: disturbances of potency, decrease in morning erections, decrease in libido and sexual activity, and 'the impression of having passed the zenith of life'. The latter is a global paraphrase and, in German, is linked to changes of sexual life for many patients, as far as we know from patients in the pre-phase of this study. The variable 'decrease in beard growth' was kept in the raw AMS scale, because experienced physicians claim that this is a symptom of severe hormonal changes that are so rare in our group of patients that the effect was diluted. For the sake of medical opinion, this symptom was kept despite the low loading.

In summary, we found three dimensions that explain most of the variance of symptoms or complaints available in the age span 40–70 years: psychological, somato-vegetative and sexual symptoms. Medical, psychosocial and other conditions clustered in other factors that are not relevant for our purposes, and were excluded from the scale.

Degenhardt and Schmidt[9] reported, from their factor analysis of the symptoms of 240 males in Germany, two factors similar to those we found: 'psychological syndrome of energy loss' and 'vegetative and vasomotor dysfunction'. They stated in their paper that sexual symptoms had no clear association with the two factors mentioned[9]. It is astonishing that very similar dimensions were also described for the MRS for women[10], which has been successfully used in medical practice to monitor hormone replacement for more than a decade.

Normal values

A representative sample of the German male population aged 40–69 years was drawn to obtain reference values for the raw AMS – that is, normal values for the severity of symptoms in each dimension of the scale for the age span under consideration. A representative population-based sample of 1000 males in this age span was drawn in Germany, and 959 questionnaires were completed. More details are published elsewhere[7].

Based on the dimensions found with factor analysis in the small but well-characterized patients group, we calculated normal values for the scores of each dimension from the answers given by the population sample. Each dimension consists of an intensity profile of a number of specific questions. Each symptom of the raw AMS scale was presented in five intensity grades: none, mild, moderate, severe and very severe. Following our general approach to developing a simple instrument for practice, we decided to add one extra scoring point with each increasing intensity grade, so that the number of scoring points for an individual question ranges from one (none) to five points (very severe). So on each question the score ranges from 1–5 points, and one dimension with five questions can score 5–25 points (cf. Figure 3: AMS scale and evaluation form).

Table 2 lists the three dimensions (subscales) of the AMS scale, reviews the symptoms that form the dimensions, and provides the minimal and maximal scores that can be obtained.

Categories of severity for the three sub-scales

For each scale, the severity of symptoms was calculated by summing the points obtained in each relevant question. Four categories (no, little, moderate and severe complaints) were distinguished. The cut-off points between the categories of the three scales were arbitrarily defined using the sum-scores to allow for an acceptable frequency distribution (many more persons with no or little complaints than severe ones). For other purposes, the continuous number of scoring points may be used or a dichotomized scale (see below) can be used.

Table 3 shows the frequency distribution of the three dimensions in the population. These

Figure 3 AMS Questionnaire

Which of the following symptoms apply to you at this time? Please, mark the appropriate box for each symptom. For symptoms that do not apply, please mark 'none'.

	Symptoms:				
	none	*mild*	*moderate*	*severe*	*extremely severe*
(Score =	1	2	3	4	5)
1. Decline in your feeling of general well-being (general state of health, subjective feeling)	☐	☐	☐	☐	☐
2. Joint pain and muscular ache (lower back pain, joint pain, pain in a limb, general back ache)	☐	☐	☐	☐	☐
3. Excessive sweating (unexpected/sudden episodes of sweating, hot flushes independent of strain)	☐	☐	☐	☐	☐
4. Sleep problems (difficulty in falling asleep, difficulty in sleeping through, waking up early and feeling tired, poor sleep, sleeplessness)	☐	☐	☐	☐	☐
5. Increased need for sleep, often feeling tired	☐	☐	☐	☐	☐
6. Irritability (feeling aggressive, easily upset about little things, moody)	☐	☐	☐	☐	☐
7. Nervousness (inner tension, restlessness, feeling fidgety)	☐	☐	☐	☐	☐
8. Anxiety (feeling panicky)	☐	☐	☐	☐	☐
9. Physical exhaustion/lacking vitality (general decrease in performance, reduced activity, lacking interest in leisure activities, feeling of getting less done, of achieving less; of having to force oneself to undertake activities)	☐	☐	☐	☐	☐
10. Decrease in muscular strength (feeling of weakness)	☐	☐	☐	☐	☐
11. Depressive mood (feeling down, sad, on the verge of tears, lack of drive, mood swings, feeling nothing is of any use)	☐	☐	☐	☐	☐
12. Feeling that you have passed your peak	☐	☐	☐	☐	☐
13. Feeling burnt out, having hit rock-bottom	☐	☐	☐	☐	☐
14. Decrease in beard growth	☐	☐	☐	☐	☐
15. Decrease in ability/frequency to perform sexually	☐	☐	☐	☐	☐
16. Decrease in the number of morning erections	☐	☐	☐	☐	☐
17. Decrease in sexual desire/libido (lacking pleasure in sex, lacking desire for sexual intercourse)	☐	☐	☐	☐	☐

Have you got any other major symptoms?   Yes ☐   No ☐
If Yes, please describe:

THANK YOU VERY MUCH FOR YOUR COOPERATION

continued

Figure 3 AMS Rating Scale evaluation form (this form explains how the total sum-score and the sum-scores of the subscales are determined)

Question Number	Score	Psychological Subscale	Somatic Subscale	Sexual Subscale
1			⟶	
2			⟶	
3			⟶	
4			⟶	
5			⟶	
6		⟶		
7		⟶		
8		⟶		
9			⟶	
10			⟶	
11		⟶		
12				⟶ ......
13		⟶		
14				⟶ ......
15				⟶ ......
16				⟶ ......
17				⟶ ......
Sum of scores in sub-scales		Sum-score PSYCH	Sum-score SOMAT	Sum-score SEXUAL ....

Total sum of scores of all subscales = Total score:

Table 2 Description of the scoring points in the three dimensions of the AMS scale. Between brackets in the column 'dimensions' are the minimal and maximal values of scoring points that can be achieved. The numbers in the 'symptoms' column reflect the number of the items in the AMS scale (cf. Figure 3)

Dimensions	Symptoms (item number)
Psychological symptoms (min: 5; max: 25 points)	irritable(6); nervous(7); anxious(8); depressive(11); burned out(13)
Somato-vegetative symptoms (min: 7; max: 35 points)	impaired well-being(1); joint and muscle complaints(2); sweating(3); sleep disturbances(4); need for more sleep(5); exhaustion(9); weakness(10)
Sexual symptoms (min: 5; max: 25 points)	Have passed peak of life (12); decrease in beard growth(14); disturbed potency(15); impaired erectile function(16); problems with libido(17)

categories can be used as reference values for observations in patients according to the German population sample.

Using a large, random population sample of German males in this age group, we could define reference values for the classification of symptom severity in each of the three dimensions, and prepare the final AMS scale.

When a summary score of the AMS is available for an individual patient, it can now be determined whether his complaints are severe, moderate, mild or not different from the normal population over 40 years of age, and also specified in three dimensions. The comparative classification of patients no longer depends on the experience of the

Table 3 Reference scores derived from the population sample of 959 males[7]. Classification of men according to four categories of symptom severity, for the total score and in the three dimensions respectively. The cut-off points for severity were defined with the initial factor analysis of the patient's group ($n = 116$). Missing information in single questions was replaced by imputation using regression analysis.

Total sum-score

Points	Impairment	n	Percent of the population
0–26	no	447	45.2
27–36	little	361	36.5
37–49	moderate	111	11.2
50+	severe	71	7.1

Psychological factor

Points	Impairment	n	Percent of the population
0–5	no	417	43.6
6–8	little	400	41.8
9–11	moderate	104	10.9
12+	severe	35	3.7

Somato-vegetative factor

Points	Impairment	n	Percent of the population
0–8	no	319	33.3
9–12	little	377	39.3
13–18	moderate	201	21
19+	severe	62	6.4

Sexual symptoms

Points	Impairment	n	Percent of the population
0–5	no	427	44.5
6–7	little	266	27.7
8–10	moderate	208	21.7
11+	severe	58	6.1

physician but on reference values obtained from the population, therefore complaints can be compared among patients treated in different medical settings.

We have no clear evidence that the sum-scores of persons aged 45–50 differ substantially from those aged 51–70 years, i.e. in this narrow age band. However, this needs be confirmed in additional investigations.

If it is desired to have more clinically based categories, the following proposal can be made: the AMS total sum-scores can be divided into three categories, which are arbitrarily defined according to the frequency distribution but not validated yet (Table 4):

(1) Normal aging – no further activities proposed (sum-score < 25);

(2) Equivocal symptoms' profile – more close (diagnostic?) observation or interventional measures (sum-score 25–44); and

(3) Important symptoms – intervention desirable; further diagnostics? (sum-score 45+)

These statistical cut-off points need to be empirically justified or modified in interven-

Table 4 AMS total sum-scores in three categories, which were arbitrarily cut into three 'clinical categories' according to the frequency distribution. For the meaning of the categories, refer to text.

This is a theoretical proposal based on statistical cut-off points which need to be empirically justified or modified in intervention studies.

Categories	Range of scores	Percent of the population
Normal aging	0–24	35
Equivocal symptoms' profile	25–45	55
Important symptoms	45–85	10

tion studies. This would also be interesting for the three sub-scales, which may be differently sensitive for hormonal intervention.

Summarizing, AMS is mainly a QoL scale, specific for aging males and not intended for use as an instrument to screen aging males for hormone deficiency – although some correlation to hormone levels may exist. But QoL is a very complex construct tied in with psychological, social, behavioral and biological patterns. Usually, scales of QoL do not show a high correlation with so-called objective (for example biological) parameters because of the complexity of the relationship. It does not mean that an intermediate relationship can be excluded, for example through symptoms of a 'relative' hormone deficiency, symptoms that are very complex in nature as well as causality. The situation in women with 'menopause scales' is similar, although the sharp decline in estrogen level is different to males. However, direct correlations among repeatedly measured scores of a menopausal scale and the hormone level may not be impressive either, both intra- and inter-individually. Comparative studies in males and females would be interesting.

STEPS TOWARD CROSS-CULTURAL VALIDATION OF THE AMS SCALE

As a first step, translation for English-speaking cultures was planned, specifically for use in the United Kingdom and North America. The procedure and results were published elsewhere[11].

Although an English version of the AMS was initially published, it was a simple word-by word translation, and was not formally validated as to whether the questions were understood in the same way as by native German speakers. It was, therefore, unclear if the same answer reflected the same content. Because conceptual rather than literal similarity is required, the translation process should guarantee that specific words and phrases reflect the culture in the respective countries.

Therefore, a linguistic and cultural translation was performed in accordance with international recommendations[12] (scheme in Figure 4):

Forward translation: into English (American and British separately, and if possible also as a uniform version). Two experienced translators, one of them the coordinator, carried out the independent translations. They kept a log of items that caused problems, and of what kind. The items were ranked according to problems with compatibility with German, when necessary taking notes of alternative phrasing with similar content if a direct translation was difficult due to different cultural backgrounds. The coordinator compared both versions and distinguished the differences.

Quality control: the coordinator arranged a personal meeting of the two translators to discuss the proposals item by item in order to find a consensus. Cultural, linguistic, emotional and other aspects were discussed to arrive at a third version. Although differences between the British and American version were identified, after comprehensive discussions it was decided to use a common version, because the differences were minor and so many 'Americanisms' are well-spread throughout Europe. This version was accepted for further work-up. Minutes were kept of the meeting and the revision process so that the

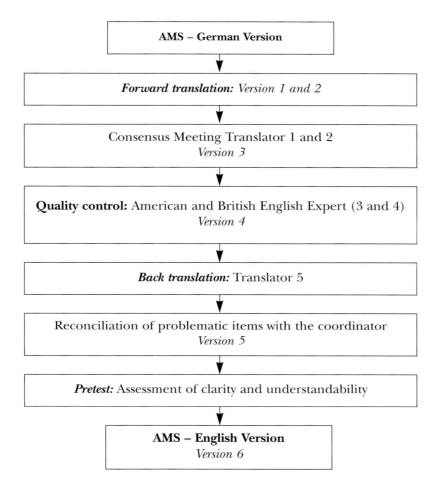

Figure 4 Procedure of linguistic and cultural validation of the AMS scale (original German) into English (British and American)

development of the revised common version three could be traced.

Two bilingual medical experts (one for British and one for American English) compared version three with the German standard and gave written assessments of the accuracy of the translation in three categories as very good, good to moderate and less satisfactory. For both latter categories, the reviewers were asked to offer alternatives. Review and subsequent verbal discussion resulted in a version four.

Backward translation: another bilingual translator, who was not involved previously, was asked to back-translate version four into German. Thereafter the translators discussed with the coordinator every discrepancy and decided whether it was a matter of content or just playing with words. Back-translation showed that the English version four was highly compatible with the German version, and changes were not required. This version can be found in Figure 3.

Pretest: prior to a broader application, a group of 22 subjects in the UK (45–65 years old and from different social backgrounds) was asked to give their opinions about understandability and clarity of the questions on a provided form and to make suggestions as to how to improve the wording of the items of the questionnaire. In addition, they answered the questionnaire twice at an interval of two to three weeks. As a result of the comments of the subjects, four items have been changed.

Recently, a similar validation of the AMS scale was completed for Dutch and French language (personal communication Julie Rambotham, MAPI Institute, Lyon, France) and for Spanish (personal communication Eric Myon, Pierre-Fabre, France), and will be published soon. Furthermore, translations also exist for Finnish, Russian, and Flemish language, but were not done in the standardized procedure described above.

Since normal values are only available from a population sample in Germany, a repetition of a population survey for each new culture to compare the reference values should be aimed for. These values will possibly not substantially deviate from the German ones, but it might be important to have evidence for this assumption. This should be done in the near future.

RESULTS OF TEST–RETEST RELIABILITY OF THE AMS SCORES

Currently, results of repeated application of the AMS scale are available for Germany and UK. The questionnaire was applied to men aged 45–65 years twice after an interval of about 14 days. This time interval was chosen as a compromise – to prevent changes of the situation/condition but also limit the impact of direct recall of the answers of the first inquiry.

The correlation between the first and second application was sufficiently high. The correlation coefficient of the total score ranged around $r = 0.9$ (UK: $r = 0.92$; GER: $r = 0.86$). Figures 5 and 6 show the scattergrams for the total scores for Germany and UK.

A Finnish research group reported from their large investigation on symptoms and hormone levels in aging males – including the

AMS scale as well as their own scales – that the test–retest reliability of the AMS is high: $r = 0.6$ ($n = 208$) and $r = 0.8$ ($n = 89$) in two subsequent years.

Together, these results point to promisingly good test characteristics of the AMS scale. However, evidence has to be provided that this is also true for other cultures. Priority is suggested for investigations under British and North American conditions (or even distinguishing between USA and Canada due to slightly different languages and cultural mix). Sample sizes of about 100 would be proposed.

Comparison with other symptom scales for aging males

The Finnish research group found a strong and statistically significant correlation of the total score of their Turku 14-item scale and the AMS scale ($r = 0.8$; $n = 95$). In other words, the two scales can be regarded as measuring the same phenomena. Moreover, the Finnish group compared all items of the AMS scale with the total score of their very short questionnaire (three items) and found statistically significant correlation coefficients ranging from 0.2–0.6 (sample size over 200) for all AMS items. Again, this speaks in favor of good test characteristics of the AMS scale.

There are other questionnaires for aging males based on symptoms/complaints, for example the Androgen Deficiency in Aging Males (ADAM) questionnaire of St. Louis University[13] and the Massachusetts Male Aging Study (MMAS) screener[14]. These two instruments were developed mainly to screen for persons with androgen deficiency associated with a symptom complex. The ADAM questionnaire consists of ten questions, whose content is similar to those of the AMS scale. The concept of this instrument, however, is different from that of the AMS and not based on a formal test construction theory. In a few persons ($n = 34$) the test–retest variation was shown (coefficient of variation 11.5%). Most importantly, a correlation of the test results with bio-available testosterone was found, and also a response of ADAM to testosterone replacement ($n = 15$) reported. Scoring and evaluation of the scale is

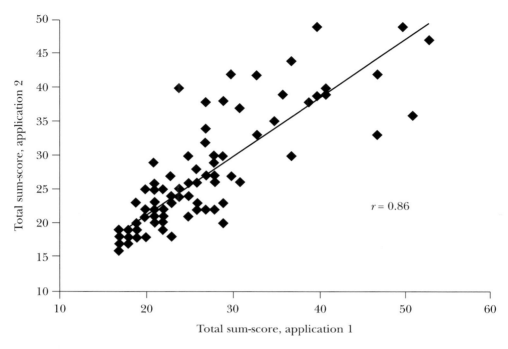

Figure 5 Test–retest reliability of the German AMS scale after an interval of two weeks in males aged 45–65 years ($n = 102$)

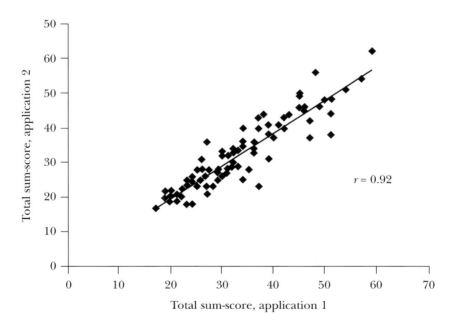

Figure 6 Test–retest reliability of the English AMS scale in males aged 45–65 years ($n = 92$)

easy, but the (population) normal distribution of the test scores is not published.

The MMAS screening test followed a broader approach: all kinds of symptoms, complaints and conditions that could be related to testosterone deficiency were included in the investigation. Thirty-four dichotomized variables of the current condition were compared to testosterone level. Those were selected for the screener that had the closest statistical association with androgen deficiency (logistic regression and factor analysis). Stepwise, eight variables were finally selected for the screening instrument as 'predictors of testosterone deficiency'. Variables of this self-administered eight-item screener got different weights. The normal distribution of the scores in the population was not reported. About 6% false negative and roughly 37% false positive test results were reported for the screener referral status. This screener was developed to motivate men with high scores to seek medical advice. In other words, the latter two instruments were primarily designed to make men aware that their symptoms could be caused by androgen deficiency, i.e. relevant for a small subgroup of aging males, and not to measure QoL of aging males in general, which may be at least partly due to relative androgen deficiency.

In fact, the comparison with other scales with similar purpose is the most important approach for validation. It is known from other QoL scales that comparisons with scales with similar purposes are much more important than comparisons with so-called objective parameters such as exercise test, physiological or chemical parameters – in our case with hormones. QoL should be validated against QoL measured with other generic or specific instruments. The results from the Finnish group are an example of a comparison with QoL scales supposed to be specific for the aging male. An example of a comparison with a generic QoL scale follows below.

AMS SCALE – COMPARISON WITH A GENERIC QUALITY OF LIFE SCALE (SF36)

The AMS scale and the SF36 questionnaire were used at the same time in 116 males aged 40–70 without serious health problems. The total score and the three sub-scores of the AMS scale were compared to sub-scales of SF36.

The AMS total sum-score and the somatic and psychologic sub-scales of SF36 were statistically significantly correlated: $r = -0.49$ ($n = 116$; $p < 0.0001$). The specific somatic and psychologic sub-scales of both instruments (AMS and SF36) are also strongly correlated, but there is no comparator for the sexual subscale of AMS in SF36. The correlation of the somato-vegetative sum-score of AMS and the somatic sum-score of SF36 can be seen in Figure 7 ($r = -0.54$; $p < 0.0001$; $n = 116$). The correlation is inverse due to the fact that the sum-scores of the AMS increase with numbers (intensity) of symptoms/complaints and the sum-scores of SF36 increase with increasing well-being/happiness.

The same applies to the correlation of the psychologic sum-scores of both instruments, which is somewhat lower – see scattergram in Figure 8 ($r = -0.65$; $p < 0.0001$; $n = 116$). The sizes of the circles in the scattergrams of both figures indicate the respective number of people.

To learn more about the correlation between the AMS sum-score and the sub-scales of SF36, we analyzed to what extent the mean values of the eight scales of SF36 differ among the quartiles of the total sum-score of AMS (Figure 9). The biggest differences were found regarding the physical (RP) and emotional role (RE), while the smallest variation was observed regarding social functioning. But the general feature is that lower quartiles of AMS sum-scores are associated with a much better profile of QoL than higher AMS sum-scores, which are indicative of many 'adropausal' symptoms.

ATTEMPTS TO EXTERNALLY VALIDATE THE AMS SCALE

Clinical opinion

We performed a comparison with one external criterion: judgment of the clinical likelihood of 'males' climacteric' according to an expert

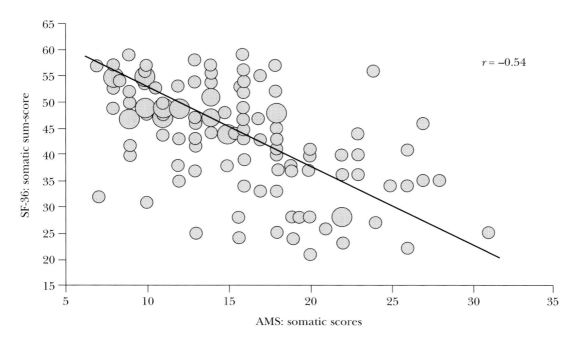

Figure 7   Correlation between somatic sum-scores of AMS scale and of the generic QoL scale SF36. The scaling towards worse quality is inverse in both scales – hence the negative correlation coefficient

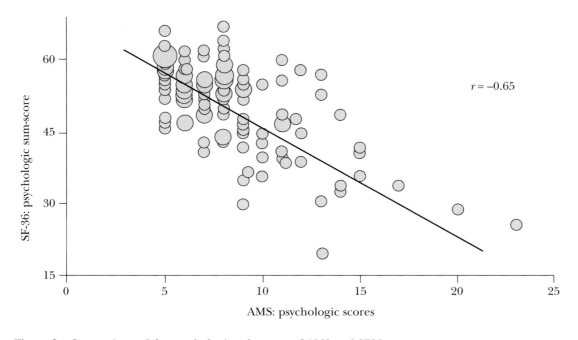

Figure 8   Comparison of the psychologic sub-scores of AMS and SF36

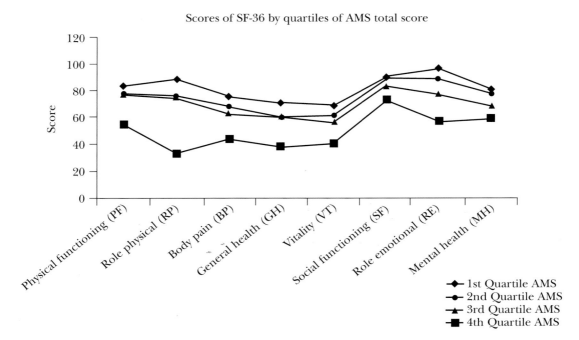

Figure 9 All sub-scales of SF36 are depicted by quartiles of the AMS total sum-score to demonstrate that the SF36 behaves similarly across the whole distribution of the AMS scale

opinion, which is a construct itself. A medical expert assessed the likelihood that the male climacteric might have started to develop for each individual person of the initial group of patients ($n = 116$). This judgment was entirely based on clinical grounds (blinded to hormone data), i.e. only using the data of the questionnaire: individual profile of symptoms, history of medical conditions (including treatment), stress situations and other lifestyle problems. It might be debatable if this can be regarded as a step of validation.

The assessment process consisted of two phases: (1) the expert read all patients' files carefully to set up and adjust his own 'internal measurement scale'; thereafter, (2) patients were classified into three groups of probability of male climacteric – likely, equivocal or unlikely. No scheme was provided to the expert as to how to assess the probability of climacteric – it was left to his clinical experience ('internal measurement scale'). The two extreme categories (likely and unlikely) were used as external criteria of

comparison with the three dimensions of the AMS scale. The middle group, where an allocation to one of the extreme groups was equivocal for the expert, was excluded from this analysis (about 35% of the 116 patients). The excluded 'equivocal group' did not clearly vary regarding the severity score in any of the three dimensions (data not shown). Table 5 shows the frequencies of the sum scores in the three dimensions and the two extreme groups of clinical probability of 'male's climacteric' (likely versus unlikely).

The scores for the dimensions 'psychological' (five questions), 'somatic' (seven questions), and 'sexual symptoms' (five questions) differed significantly among the two extreme groups of clinical likelihood of male climacteric (chi-square test). It was pronounced most strongly in the dimension 'sexual symptoms' and less so for 'psychological symptoms'. We found a tendency in each of the AMS dimensions for the proportion of patients with 'likely male climacteric' to increase with ascending severity

Table 5 Severity of symptoms in the three AMS dimensions and probability of the clinical diagnosis 'male climacteric'. Only the two extreme groups were used for this tabulation, i.e. where the clinical judgment was unequivocal, either 'likely' or 'unlikely'. (Out of 116 patients, 76 could be classified; in 40 the expert arrived at no clear decision and this subgroup was dropped in this table.)
The numbers available for analysis differ among the dimensions due to missing information. Chi-square test was applied to test for significant differences in severity of symptoms between the two groups (p-values).

| | | Male climacteric (clinical judgment) | | |
	n (total)	Likely n (%)	Unlikely n (%)	p
Psychological symptoms				
no	12	6 (50)	6 (50)	
little	32	16 (50)	16 (50)	
moderate	14	13 (93)	1 (7)	
severe	9	7 (78)	2 (22)	0.02
Somato-vegetative symptoms				
no or little*	35	15 (43)	20 (57)	
moderate	27	23 (85)	4 (15)	
severe	14	12 (86)	2 (14)	0.0005
Sexual symptoms				
no or little*	29	5 (17)	24 (83)	
moderate	21	20 (95)	1 (5)	
severe	25	24 (96)	1 (4)	0

*Two categories were combined because one cell was zero

of scores, whereas it decreased in the group where male climacteric was deemed unlikely by clinical judgment.

The obvious problems besides small numbers of patients in the two extreme groups are that we cannot validate the validation criterion 'clinical probability of male climacteric' and that clinical climacteric symptoms need not necessarily find their expression in hormone values. In other words, it is a very weak piece of information. We have to accumulate further evidence that the AMS scale really measures a male climacteric-related phenomenon (construct validation). There is currently no simple gold standard for the clinical definition of 'male climacteric'.

Correlation of AMS with hormone levels

As mentioned earlier already, it is doubtful whether correlations with hormone levels are a realistic goal. It is unlikely that a QoL scale correlates significantly with the profile of hormones. However, if many hormones are tested, one significant correlation might appear just due to multiple testing. QoL is a subjective expression of a network of somatic and psychic functions, and hormone levels influence these functions through various channels. Hormone levels and QoL, however, are different levels in reality.

Nevertheless, we measured some hormone values and observed no important correlations with the sum-scores of the AMS or any of the subscales for the total group of patients ($n = 116$). The analysis of specific subgroups of patients with or without signs of deficiency of testosterone or 17β-estradiol in serum showed that there was an impact on the prevalence of severe symptoms – at least to some extent. Sexual symptoms tend to be more frequent in the group with real testosterone and/or estradiol deficiency compared with the group of physiological hormone levels (Figure 10).

It would be helpful for a better understanding of the AMS scale to show if a relevant hormonal intervention will find its expression also in changes of AMS scores. Such studies are

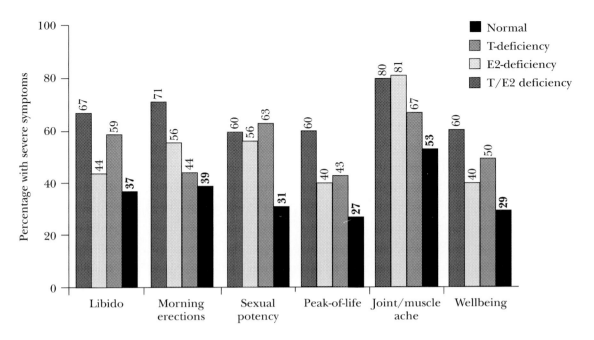

Figure 10 Frequency of severe complaints (variables of the AMS) in males with normal testosterone and estradiol levels (normal; $n = 48$), with deficiency of free testosterone but normal estradiol (T; $n = 29$), deficiency of estradiol (E2; $n = 16$), or deficiency of both testosterone & estradiol (T/E2; $n = 15$). Most other items of the AMS showed no associations with hormones

in preparation and would definitely contribute to the construct validity (stepwise construct validation of the term 'males' climacteric' and the AMS scale) and to the development of the AMS scale as a follow-up instrument for clinical practice.

NEED FOR FURTHER RESEARCH

Although the AMS scale is already a stand-ardized instrument to measure QoL aspects for aging males with much empirical information available, there are still many loose ends. The cross-cultural validation needs to be completed, particularly for Spanish – at least from the European and Latin American perspective. In the same context, attempts are needed to confirm normal values for the scores in cultures other than German. Even

small studies would be helpful to gain an impression of whether the variation among cultures is high or not important.

Furthermore, it is necessary to learn how closely related the AMS scores are with hormonal intervention (for instance, andro-gens, estrogens, or growth hormone) in real practice. The question is: to what extent do the AMS sum-scores vary pre/post-intervention and to what extent is the variation related to the subjective overall assessment of the treatment effect?

An objective for the more distant future is to understand what the AMS scale is measuring. First of all this is a theoretical question to be answered by means of construct validation. But it also has practical implications: it might be possible to develop more-specific instruments.

References

1. Werner AA. The male climacteric: report of 273 cases. *J Am Med Assoc* 1946;132:188–94
2. Bauer J. The male climacteric – a misnomer. *J Am Med Assoc* 1944;126:914–18
3. Degenhardt A. Wechseljahre beim Mann, gibt es sie? In: Fischer S, Streb-Lieder, Vogt, eds. *Wechseljahre für Fortgeschrittene.* Frankfurt:Verlag für Akademische Schriften, 1995:104–18
4. McKinlay JB, Longcope CH, Gray A. The questionable physiological and epidemiologic basis for a male climacteric syndrome: preliminary results from the Massachusetts Male Aging Study. *Maturitas* 1989;11:103–5
5. Kupperman HS, Blatt MHG, Wiesbaden H, *et al.* Comparative clinical evaluation of estrogen preparations by the menopausal and amenorrhoeal indices. *J Clin Endocrinol* 1953;13:88–95
6. Hauser GA, Huber IC, Keller PJ, *et al.* Evaluation der klimakterischen Beschwerden (Menopause Rating Scale (MRS). *Zentralbl Gynakol* 1994;116:16–23
7. Heinemann LAJ, Zimmermann T, Vermeulen A, *et al.* A New 'Aging Male's Symptoms' (AMS) Rating Scale. *Aging Male* 1999;2:105–114
8. Heinemann LAJ, Thiel C, Assmann A, *et al.* Sex differences of 'climacteric symptoms' with increasing age. A hypothesis-generating analysis of cross-sectional population surveys. *The Aging Male* 2000;3:124–131
9. Degenhardt A, Schmidt H. Physische Leistungsvariablen als Indikatoren für die Diagnose 'Klimakterium Virile'. *Sexuologie* 1994;3:131–41
10. Potthoff P, Heinemann LAJ, Schneider HPG, *et al.* Menopause-Rating-Skala (MRS II): Methodische Standardisierung in der deutschen Bevölkerung. *Zentralbl Gynaekol* 2000;122:280–6
11. Heinemann LAJ, Saad F, Thiele K, *et al.* The aging males symptoms (AMS) rating scale cultural and linguistic validation into English. *Aging Male* 2001;4:14–22
12. Anonymous. Trust introduces new translation criteria. Medical Outcomes Trust Bulletin 1997;5:2–4
13. Morley JE, Charlton E, Patrick P, *et al.* Validation of a screening questionnaire for androgen deficiency in aging males. *Metabolism* 2000;49:1239–42
14. Smith KW, Feldman HA, McKinlay JB. Construction and field validation of a self-administered screener for testosterone deficiency (hypogonadism) in aging men. *Clin Endocrinol* 2000;53:703–11

Psychosocial factors associated with the use of hormone replacement therapy

6

A. Collins and B.-M. Landgren

OPPOSING MODELS OF MENOPAUSE

In recent years there has been a marked upsurge of interest in women's health at menopause. Biomedical research dominates the field. Since it is ultimately up to women to decide about their own health, it is important to understand the different factors that influence women's experiences. Psychosocial scientists have pointed out that the experience of menopause is profoundly influenced by women's perception of bodily changes and their perception of how menopause is viewed in their particular society[1-3]. However, controversy and polarization of views still fuel the debate over how best to conceptualize the menopausal experience of women. The biomedical model of menopause has focused on the biological aspects of declining hormonal levels and on identifying symptoms of the climacteric syndrome. Menopause is thus characterized as a deficiency disease requiring treatment and the treatment is hormone replacement therapy (HRT), making patients out of healthy women, since symptoms are believed to be directly linked to estrogen deficiency. It should be emphasized that the only symptoms that have been directly associated with decreasing estrogen levels are night sweats and hot flushes[4]. Management of the menopause is one of the most controversial issues in medical practice today since there are a multitude of different interventions available.

Women increasingly face conflicting images of menopause and thus decisions about treatment in the context of different ideologies[5]. Several critics have asserted that the biomedical model is negative and largely determines how women view themselves, and how they are seen in society. This may lead to medicalization, leaving menopausal women dependent on the medical establishment to manage their health. Women may feel that they are not in control of their own health and have to seek medical advice in order to be diagnosed as menopausal[6,7]. Medical control of women in the menopause can be extended by playing on women's fears of aging and for their health as they age[8]. Advertisements and the media are also portraying the image of the menopause as a condition that needs intervention and treatment. Gannon and Stevens[9] found that the medical model of menopause was used in media to convey information about menopause. It is also pointed out that the biomedical model is largely based on data collected from clinical populations that are not representative of women in general, the results of which are then generalized to all women, creating a biased view[10]. Morse and colleagues[11] found that treatment-seeking women differed from other women in their self-concept and earlier treatment-seeking behavior.

Social scientists, on the other hand, have emphasized the social and cultural construct of menopause, describing menopause as a natural event and a life transition requiring adaptation and psychosocial change. Whether climacteric symptoms are experienced, and the intensity of these, is associated with the meaning attached to menopause in a particular society, and the different roles that women occupy, as well as perception of these roles. According to the socio-cultural model, it is the meaning given to menopause and to being an older woman in a particular society that will influence women's experience of menopause. The value of and the attitudes towards women, and the role of women in midlife, may influence the experience of menopause[1,12]. The psychosocial meaning of menopause also plays a vital role in the decision of whether or not to start HRT[13]. The perception of menopause as a medical condition correlates significantly with HRT use, transforming healthy women into patients and rendering them dependent on health care services. On the other hand, social and cultural attitudes to menopause may also prevent women who could benefit from HRT from seeking medical attention and receiving treatment.

More recent trends in epidemiological research have highlighted the need to integrate these two opposing views into a more holistic, interactive model that takes into account more complex and multifaceted aspects of menopause. Flint[14] suggested a psycho-bio-cultural model of menopause for interdisciplinary research and for a better understanding of the different aspects of women's health. Olazabal and colleagues[5] have suggested a more holistic approach to menopause, a more balanced view.

INTENTIONS TO USE OR NOT USE HRT

Hormone replacement is being promoted for the relief of vasomotor symptoms and the prevention of osteoporosis and cardiovascular disease, and prevention of Alzheimer's disease. New evidence is being generated regarding the benefits and risks, and currently it is not clear whether the previously held opinion that estrogen treatment has secondary preventive effect on coronary artery disease[15] holds true. To date, there is strong evidence that estrogen treatment prevents bone loss during the early postmenopausal years[16]. However, the evidence for HRT in the prevention of fractures is weaker[17]. HRT is also being promoted for improvement in quality of life and for mood changes, but the evidence is clearly very contradictory. Whether women are able to

Table 1 Reasons for starting hormone replacement therapy

Reason	Percentage of women giving reason
Relief from physical symptoms	74
Relief from psychological symptoms	14
Prevention of disease	6
To keep young	6

assess their future risk of disease is not quite clear. Hunter and co-workers[18] found that mid-age women tended to have a reasonably accurate perception of their future risk of developing diseases such as heart disease and osteoporosis, although they tended to over-estimate the risk of breast cancer.

When asked for reasons for starting HRT, women in our longitudinal study[19] responded with relief from physical symptoms (74%), relief from psychological symptoms (14%), prevention of disease (6%) and to keep young (6%) (Table 1). Similar results were reported by Kaufert and colleagues[20]. Ambivalent feelings and thoughts were reported to be related to fears of side-effects such as irregular menstruation and fear of cancer. Fear of cancer, particularly breast cancer, was reported by Schneider and co-workers[21] and Vihtamäki and colleagues[22] as very strongly related to not starting or discontinuing HRT. Countless studies have reported a high rate of discontinuation, and it seems that more than 50% of women who start HRT discontinue treatment after the first year or earlier[23]. The medical literature deals extensively with the problem of compliance in terms of uptake and adherence to treatment regimens. Low compliance is seen mainly as a problem of inadequate information. There are several studies of the role of knowledge, counseling strategies and how best to inform women of the benefits as well as the risks of HRT.

WOMEN'S VIEWS OF HRT

Recently, much research has focused on how midlife women construct their own menopausal experience[24–26]. Woods and colleagues[25] found different themes in women's experiences. Most women did not refer to menopause as a time of loss but spoke of menopause as a time of symptoms, changing emotions, hormonal change, a changing body and the aging process. However, menopause as a time of disease risk or increased need for medical attention was infrequently mentioned. Woods and co-workers concluded that women's views had not been influenced by the medical definition of menopause. Jones showed in a small qualitative study[26] that many women had ambivalent feelings of being treated with HRT. These studies showed that women's models of menopause did not reflect the definition of menopause as a medical event. Hunter and colleagues, in their study[24], also found that women resisted the medical model and saw menopause in terms of a developmental phase that does not need medical intervention.

In fact, there is evidence from interview studies that women are increasingly taking control of their own decisions and that they are resisting medicalization[8,24,26]. Women are not merely passive consumers but are developing critical thinking and are questioning their doctors' advice to start and to maintain HRT. Interestingly, women who made their own decision to initiate HRT were more likely to continue treatment. Our results also suggest that it may be important that women feel it is their own decision. More women who reported that the doctor had initiated treatment discontinued HRT within three years compared with those who said that they themselves had initiated HRT[27]. The decision to take HRT is complex, as Lewis[28] points out, since the risks and benefits associated with it are uncertain. Many women who are taking HRT have many unanswered questions about treatment and want to know more about the benefits and side-effects, particularly the long-term side-effects. Griffith[8] emphasized that it is a dynamic process and that women are continually re-assessing their situation when new knowledge is available.

Other studies have focused on how women obtain information and collect their knowl-edge, how they make their decision to start HRT or not and what processes ensue when they start therapy. Lauver and colleagues[29] and Hunter et al[18] pointed out that women's preferences for HRT use may be based on short-term effects (such as relief of symptoms), fear of side-effects and personal attitude whereas clinicians and researchers recommend HRT based on long-term gains, with a population focus. A Canadian study[30] showed that perceived health benefits and social support from significant others, and not perceived side-effects, were the most important predictors of women's use of HRT. Armstrong and co-workers[31], in a recent study, showed that the fear of breast cancer was not a significant factor in womem's decision making. From women's perspective, their feelings, beliefs and decisions should be respected by the health care providers regardless of the recommendations of medical research[32]. Research findings are beginning to show how women arrive at their decisions. If the factors that explain women's decisions about hormone therapy were understood more fully, clinicians could integrate this knowledge and they could be more helpful in the process.

A range of psychosocial variables has been found to influence care-seeking behavior[29]. Education and socio-economic status are important variables that affect hormone use.

SOCIO-ECONOMIC AND ETHNIC DIFFERENCES

Few studies so far have evaluated the sociodemographic and psychosocial predictors of HRT use. It seems clear that there are important differences between women that predispose them to either opt for treatment or stay away from it. The advice and recommendation of doctors, particularly gynecologists, seem to be powerful predictors of HRT use[33] and studies show the use of HRT is strongly related to the interaction between women and their physicians[34]. A positive attitude and encouragement from the physician are particularly important[35] and women who see a female gynecologist are more likely to be prescribed HRT[36]. In Scandinavia, female gynecologists themselves have high rates of HRT use. In a Swedish study 88% of female gynecologists were using HRT compared to about 40% in the general population[27,37], clearly demonstrating their positive view of the treatment.

There is a significant difference in HRT use between socio-economic groups[38,39]. Women with a moderate to high income have been shown to be three times more likely to be taking HRT compared with women on a low income. Lydakis and colleagues[40] reported a higher awareness of HRT among women with a higher education. It is possible that women with a low income do not seek medical advice or do not have access to health care to the same extent as women from higher socio-economic groups. It is also possible that doctors are less likely to prescribe HRT to women of lower socio-economic status[41,42]. Recent studies have focused on the prescribing patterns of female and male gynecologists and the findings are somewhat contradictory. There are a number of studies showing that gynecologists, and particularly female gynecologists, have a higher prescription rate compared to other physicians[43,44]. However, one study[42] showed that male gynecologists spent more time counseling women and were more likely to prescribe HRT.

A bias in prescribing HRT to women has been documented. There is evidence to show that doctors are more likely to prescribe HRT to healthy women[44,45]. There are also marked differences between ethnic groups. It was shown that African-American women, although they reported more hot flushes, did not receive as much counseling for HRT as white women[46]. The African-American women were motivated to learn more and they also had a more positive attitude to menopause than white women. In a recent American study of different ethnic groups and using retrospective medical records it was found that white women were more likely to receive prescriptions for HRT than Hispanic, Asian, African-American and Soviet-immigrant women[47]. There may be cultural factors affecting the communication between the woman and the doctor. The largest disparity in the study was that between the Soviet immigrants and the other women in the study which may reflect significant cultural differences and maybe difficulties in language and the patient–physician dialogue.

INDIVIDUAL DIFFERENCES BETWEEN WOMEN

Women are very much influenced by the norms in society, by the images of menopause in the media, by their friends, and by their doctors. There are distinct differences in the duration of HRT use between women. However, research has found that long-term users are not different from short-term or non users[8,35]. Griffith[8] noted that long-term therapy for prevention of disease has not received a high priority among women.

There are several studies suggesting that a healthier lifestyle, more frequent physical exercise, a lower body-mass index, and better self-rated health is correlated with HRT use[19,44,48,49]. The results suggest that women who are already more health conscious, who exercise more frequently and eat better diets are the ones who will choose HRT. These women also go for more frequent health checks such as pap smears and mammography[27,50] and they tend to have a higher intake of alternative remedies as well as vitamins and calcium supplementation[51,52]. A recent French study[53] reported that women who were motivated to preserve their young looks and who conceived of replacement therapy as an anti-age compound were more likely to use HRT and see it as a cosmetic product. Schultz-Zehden[54], in a survey of German women, found that one reason for starting treatment was to keep their sexual attractiveness. The results also indicated differences in enduring personality traits between users and non-users, users scoring as more anxious, emotionally labile and having more traditionally feminine traits than non-users as measured by a personality inventory.

Women's social roles and employment status play a significant part in the use of HRT. Several studies have found that women who are employed and those who work full-time are more likely to be HRT users[55,56]. Our own longitudinal population-based study of transition to menopause[57] showed that women with mentally demanding work and women who thought about work in their leisure time, as well as women who reported life stress at baseline and during the previous two years, were significantly more often HRT users. In contrast, women with physically demanding work were less likely to be using HRT. Kaufert[58] has pointed out that women have to balance menopausal symptoms and work demands, and may be choosing HRT to do so. Legare and colleagues[59], in a French study using telephone interviews, found that women believed that they would perform better at work and in their relationships if they were using HRT.

CULTURAL DIFFERENCES IN THE USE OF HRT

Kaufert[60] developed a conceptual model of menopause in which there are important implications of becoming menopausal that vary between societies. The definition of menopause is derived from the meaning of menopause in that society and from how women's roles are defined in a particular society. The beliefs and expectations of the prevailing ideology provide the underlying structure for development of attitudes to menopause, which in turn influence the experience of women. Thus, of particular relevance are the beliefs, values and assumptions concerning midlife women[61]. Women are aware of these cultural stereotypes and frequently interpret their bodily changes according to what they have learned. "It will act as a filter through which physiological and psychological experiences are interpreted."[58] Different cultures have different norms for symptom expression. Access to healthcare also varies widely among countries. The developing countries and developed countries differ from one another politically, economically and socially in lifestyle, women's roles and healthcare systems. It has been emphasized that women's choices at this period of their lives will have consequences for their health

into old age. Educated women in industrialized countries with well-developed medical care have access to the most recent information on hormones whereas less privileged groups do not have the same opportunities.

Studies comparing European countries show the rate of HRT varies widely from 12% in Israel[62] and 18% in Spain to 55% in France[63]. A recent Bulgarian study[64] showed that the rate of HRT is increasing and that women showed clear benefits from treatment as far as quality of life is concerned. Even in such a homogenous region as Scandinavia, there are differences in attitudes toward HRT. In 1981 HRT use was three times more common in Denmark than in Norway[65]. In 1992 use had increased in all Scandinavian countries except for Denmark, and was highest in Finland and Sweden. Use of HRT was related to education, employment and occupational status in Finland and Sweden but not in Denmark and Norway[66]. It is interesting to note that the rate of HRT use has increased significantly in Norway over the last decade and yet educated Norwegian women, though recognizing the benefits of HRT, have proved to be the most ambivalent about using the treatment[67]. In a recent comparative study on knowledge, attitudes and management strategies concerning HRT use in Denmark, Norway and Sweden[65], 42% offered HRT to all women, provided there was no contraindication, while 58% recommended HRT to select women after considering the advantages and disadvantages of HRT. There were no differences between the three countries regarding indications and contraindications to HRT.

The most cited cross-cultural difference is that observed between Western countries and Asian countries. Japanese women do not experience the same frequency or intensity of vasomotor symptoms as women in the West[68,69]. Locke's interpretation of these data implied that the meaning of menopause is different in Japanese society and that Japanese women are more involved in their changing social roles rather than being influenced by biological changes. Another possible explanation may be that Asian women do not suffer from hot flushes to the same extent as Western women because their dietary intake is rich in phytoestrogens, which may have beneficial effects counteracting hot flushes[70]. The use of HRT is very low in Japan – 2.5% according to Nagata and colleagues[52] and 1.4% according to a review by Aso[71]. Traditionally Japanese women use alternative treatments such as herbs. However, according to a vocal critic[72], Japanese women do suffer from hot flushes, but cultural norms prevent them from expressing these symptoms. Furthermore, gynecologists are unwilling to prescribe HRT because of the lack of endorsement by government authorities.

CONCLUSIONS

According to the biomedical model of menopause, women should be treated with HRT. Psychosocial studies show that women are resisting medicalization and are trying to control their own health. The decision to start hormone therapy is a complex one, since the risks involved and the outcome are uncertain. Perceived health effects and social support, as well as physicians' positive attitude and

recommendations are powerful predictors of HRT use. The main reasons for discontinuation of treatment are side-effects such as irregular bleeding and anxiety about cancer, particularly breast cancer. There are distinct differences between individual women, with educated, employed and health-conscious women being more likely to use HRT. This self-selection for treatment is due to social factors such as education and socio-economic status, and to differential access to information and healthcare, as well as differences in prescription patterns and doctors' attitudes. There are also marked differences between ethnic groups in prescription rates and, from a global perspective, in the rates of HRT use between different countries. These differences may reflect political, social and economic factors as well as differential access to healthcare. The results underscore the importance of respecting women's feelings and beliefs, of promoting positive attitudes to midlife and of making education about HRT accessible to women of all socio-economic and ethnic groups, in order for them to make informed decisions.

References

1. Gannon K, Ekstrom B. Attitudes towards menopause. The influence of sociocultural paradigms. *Psychol Women Quart* 1993;17:275–88
2. Bell S. Sociological perspectives on the medicalization of menopause. In Flint M, Kronenberg F, Utian W, eds. *Multidisciplinary Perspectives on Menopause.* New York: The New York Academy of Sciences 1990:173–8
3. Kaufert PA, Locke M. Medicalization of women's third age. *J Psychosom Obstet Gynecol* 1997;18:81–6
4. Khan SA, Pace JE, Cox L, et al. Climacteric symptoms in healthy middle-aged women. *Br J Clin Pract* 1994;48:240–2
5. Olazabal Ulacia JC, Garcia Paniagua R, Montero Luengo J, et al. Models of intervention in menopause: proposal of a holistic or integral model. *Menopause* 1999;6:264–72
6. Hovelius B, Ekstrom H, Landgren BM, et al. Climacteric-medicalization, minimalization or normalization. *Läkartidningen* 2000;13:5927–30
7. Kaufert PA. The social and cultural context of menopause (review). *Maturitas* 1996;23:169–80
8. Griffith F. Women's control and choice regarding HRT. *Soc Sci Med* 1999;49:469–81
9. Gannon L, Stevens J. Portraits of menopause in the media. *Women Health* 1998;27:1–15
10. Ballard KD, Kuh DJ, Wadsworth MEJ. The role of menopause in women's experiences of the change of life. *Sociol Health Illn* 2001;23:397–424
11. Morse C, Smith A, Dennerstein D, et al. The treatment-seeking woman at menopause. *Maturitas* 1994;18:161–73
12. Collins A. Sociocultural issues in menopause. In Paoletti R, Wenger N, eds. *Women's Health and Menopause. A Global Approach.* National Institute of Health, in press
13. Lomranz J, Becker D, Eyal N, et al. Attitudes towards hormone replacement therapy among middle-aged women and men. *Eur J Obstet Gynecol Reprod Biol* 2000;93:199–203
14. Flint M, Samil RS. Cultural and subcultural

meanings of the menopause. *Ann NY Acad Sci* 1990;592:134–48

15. Hulley S, Grady D, Bush T, *et al.* Randomized trial of estrogen plus progestins for secondary prevention of coronary heart disease in postmenopausal women. *J Am Med Assoc* 1998; 19:605–13

16. Gallagher JC. Role of estrogens in the management of postmenopausal bone loss. *Rheum Dis Clin North Am* 2001;27:143–62

17. Salmen T, Heikkinen AM, Mahonen A, *et al.* The protective effect of hormone replacement therapy on fracture risk is modulated by estrogen receptor alpha genotype in early postmenopausal women. *J Bone Miner Res* 2000; 15:2479–86

18. Hunter M, O'Dea I. Perception of future health risks in mid-aged women: estimates with and without behavioral changes and hormone replacement therapy. *Maturitas* 1999;33:37–43

19. Barth Olofsson A, Collins A. Psychosocial factors, attitude to menopause and symptoms in Swedish perimenopausal women. *Climacteric* 2000;3:33–42

20. Kaufert P, Boggs P, Ettinger B, *et al.* Women and menopause: beliefs, attitudes and behaviors. The North American Menopause Society 1997 Survey. *Menopause* 1998;5:197–8

21. Schneider HP. HRT and cancer risk: separating fact from fiction. *Maturitas* 1999;33 Suppl 1: S65–72

22. Vihtamäki T, Suvilahti R, Tuimala R. Why do postmenopausal women discontinue hormone replacement therapy? *Maturitas* 1999;33:99–105

23. Groenevelt F, Bareman F, Barentsen R, *et al.* Determinants of first prescription of hormone replacement therapy. A follow-up study of 1689 women aged 45–60 years. *Maturitas* 1995;20: 81–9

24. Hunter M, O'Dea I, Britten N. Decision-making and hormone replacement therapy: a qualitative analysis. *Soc Sci Med* 1997;45:1541–8

25. Woods N, Saver B, Taylor T. Attitudes toward menopause and hormone therapy among women with access to health care. *Menopause* 1998;5:178–88

26. Jones JB. Representations of menopause and their health care implications: a qualitative study. *Am J Prev Med* 1999;13:58–65

27. Collins A, Landgren B.-M. Psychosocial factors associated with the use of hormonal replacement therapy in a longitudinal follow-up of Swedish women. *Maturitas* 1997;28:1–9

28. Lewis J. Feminism, the menopause and hormone replacement therapy. *Feminist Rev* 1993; 43:38–56

29. Lauver DR, Settersten L, Marten S, *et al.* Explaining women's intentions and use of hormones with menopause. *Res Nurs Health* 1999;22:309–20

30. Fisher WA, Sand M, Lewis W, *et al.* Canadian menopause study I: understanding women's intentions to utilise hormone replacement therapy. *Maturitas* 2000;37:1–14

31. Armstrong K, Popik S, Guerra C, *et al.* Beliefs about breast cancer risk and use of postmenopausal hormone replacement therapy. *Med Decis Making* 2000;20:308–13

32. Woods NF, Mitchell ES. Anticipating menopause: observations from the Seattle Midlife Women's Health Study. *Menopause* 1999;6: 167–73

33. Finley C, Gregg EW, Solomon LJ, *et al.* Disparities in hormone replacement use by socioeconomic status in a primary care population. *J Community Health* 2001;26:39–50

34. Newton KM, Lacroix AZ, Leveille S, *et al.* The physician's role in women's decision making about hormone replacement therapy. *Obstet Gynecol* 1998;92:580–4

35. Buist DS, Lacroix AZ, Newton KM, *et al.* Are long-term hormone replacement users different from short-term and never users? *Am J Epidemiol* 1999;149:275–81

36. Ettinger B, Woods N, Barrett-Connor E, *et al.* The North American Menopause Society 1998 Survey: Part II. Counseling about hormone replacement therapy: association with socioeconomic status and access to medical care. *Menopause* 2000;7:143–8

37. Andersson K, Pedersen AT, Mattsson LA, *et al.* Swedish gynecologists and general practitioners' views on the climacteric period: knowledge, attitudes and management strategies. *Acta Obstet Gynecol Scand* 1998;77:909–16

38. Chiaffarino F, Parazzani F, LaVeccchia C, *et al.* Correlates of hormone replacement therapy use in Italian women 1992–96. *Maturitas* 1999; 33:107–15

39. MacLaren A, Woods NF. Midlife women making hormone therapy decisions. *Womens Health Issues* 2001;11:216–30

40. Lydakis C, Kerr H, Hutchings K, *et al.* Women's awareness of and attitudes towards hormone replacement therapy: ethnic differences and effects of age and education. *Int Clin Pract* 1998; 52:7–12

41. Appling SE, Allen JK, Van Zandt S, *et al.* Knowledge about menopause and hormone replacement therapy use in low-income urban women. *J Womens Health Gend Based Med* 2000;9: 57–64

42. Huston S, Sleath B, Rubin RH. Physician gender and hormone replacement therapy discussion. *J Wom Health Gend Based Med* 2001; 10:279–87

43. Newton KM, LaCroix AZ, Buist DS, *et al.* What factors account for hormone replacement therapy prescribing frequency? *Maturitas* 2001; 39:1–10

44. Hemminki E, Topo P. Prescribing of hormone therapy in menopause and postmenopause. *J Psychosom Obstet Gynecol* 1997 18:145–57

45. Barrett Connor E. Postmenopausal estrogen and prevention bias. *Ann Intern Med* 1991;115:455–6

46. Pham KTC, Freeman E, Grisso JA. Menopause and hormone replacement therapy: focus groups of African American and Caucasian women. *Menopause* 1997;4:71–9

47. Brown AF, Perez Stable EJ, Whitaker EE, *et al.* Ethnic differences in hormone replacement prescribing patterns. *J Gen Intern Med* 1999;14:663–9

48. Matthews KA, Kuller LH, Wing RR, *et al.* Prior to use of estrogen replacement therapy – are users healthier than nonusers? *Am J Epidemiol* 1996;143:971–8

49. Matthews KA, Abrams B, Crawford S, *et al.* Body mass index in midlife women: relative influence of menopause, hormone use and ethnicity. *Int J Obes Relat Metab Disord* 2001;25:863–73

50. Shelley J, Smith A, Dudley E, *et al.* Use of hormone replacement therapy by Melbourne women. *Aust J Public Health* 1995;19:387–92

51. Stadberg E, Mattson LÅ, Milsom I. Factors associated with climacteric symptoms and the use of hormone replacement therapy. *Acta Obstet Scand* 2000;79:286–92

52. Nagata C, Matsushita Y, Shimizu H. Prevalence of hormone replacement therapy and user's characteristics: a community survey in Japan. *Maturitas* 1996;25:201–7

53. Fauconnier A, Ringa V, Delanoe D, *et al.* Use of hormone replacement therapy: women's representations of menopause and beauty care practices. *Maturitas* 2000;35:215–28

54. Schultz-Zehden B. Hormone replacement therapy – women's expectations and fears. *Z Arztl Fortbild Qual* 2000;94:180–8

55. Li C, Samsioe G, Lidfelt J, *et al.* Important factors for use of hormone replacement therapy: A population-based study of Swedish women. *Menopause* 2000;7:273–81

56. France K, Schofield MJ, Lee C. Patterns and correlates of hormone replacement therapy use in middle-aged Australian women. *Womens Health* 1997;3:121–38

57. Barth Olofsson A, Collins A. Psychosocial characteristics of Swedish women using hormone replacement therapy. Poster presented at the 9th International Menopause Congress in Yokohama, October 2000

58. Kaufert PA. A health and social profile of the menopausal woman. *Exp Gerontol* 1994;29:343–50

59. Legare F, Godin G, Guilbert E, *et al.* Determinants of the intention to adopt hormone replacement therapy among premenopausal women. *Maturitas* 2000;34:211–18

60. Kaufert PA. Myth and the menopause. *Sociol Health Illn* 1982;4:141–66

61. Bowles CL. The menopausal experience. Sociocultural influences and theoretical models. In Formanek R, ed. *The Meaning of Menopause. Historical and Clinical Perspectives.* Hillsdale: The Analytic Press, 1990:157–75

62. Blumberg G, Kaplan B, Rabinerson D, *et al.* Women's attitudes towards menopause and hormone replacement therapy. *Int J Gynaecol Obstet* 1996;54:271–7

63. Schneider HPG. Cross-national study of women's use of hormone replacement therapy (HRT) in Europe. *Int J Fertil Womens Med* 1997; Suppl 2:365–75

64. Borissova AM, Kovatcheva R, Shinkov A, *et al.* A study of the psychological status and sexuality in middle-aged Bulgarian women: significance of the hormone replacement therapy (HRT). *Maturitas* 2001;39:177–83

65. Nilsen ST, Pedersen A, Moen MH, *et al.* Knowledge, attitudes and management strategies in Scandinavia concerning hormone replacement therapy. A comparison between gynecologists in Denmark, Norway and Sweden. *Maturitas* 2001; 39:83–90

66. Topo P, Koster A, Holte A, *et al.* Trends in the use of climacteric hormones in Nordic countries. *Maturitas* 1995;22:89–95

67. Sogaard AJ, Tollan A, Berntsen GKR, *et al.* Hormone replacement therapy: Knowledge, attitudes, self-reported use – and sales figures in Nordic women. *Maturitas* 2000;35:201–14

68. Locke MM. Ambiguities of aging: Japanese experience and perceptions of menopause. *Cult Med Psychiatry* 1986;10:23–46

69. Locke MM. Menopause: lessons from anthropology (review). *Psychosom Med* 1998;60:410–19

70. Eden J. Phytoestrogens and the menopause (review). *Baillieres Clin Endocrinol Metab* 1998;12:581–7

71. Aso T. The significance of the menopause in human life in the present and the next centuries. In Aso T, Fujimoto S, eds. *The Menopause at the New Millennium.* London: Parthenon Publishing, 2000:88–94

72. Albery N. The menopause in Japan – Konenki Jigoku (editorial). *Climacteric* 1999;2:160–1

Depressed mood during the menopause transition: a review of longitudinal studies

7

A. M. Mariella and N. Fugate Woods

INTRODUCTION

As the population of US baby boomers move into their middle years, investigators and clinicians alike have focused their attention on understanding menopause and its relationship to health. One question of special interest to women has been whether depression is related to menopause. In particular, women whose mothers became depressed during midlife or women who have had previous experiences with depression express concern about their own menopausal experiences[1]. Contemporary work has left the question of the relationship of menopause to depression unanswered.

DEPRESSED MOOD AND DEPRESSION: DEFINITIONS

One of the challenges in comparing the results of studies of longitudinal patterns of depression in midlife women is the lack of clarity of the definitions related to both depression and menopause. Depression is a general term[2], usually measured in longitudinal studies by rating symptoms with respect to severity, duration and course. Depressive symptoms, such as negative affect, somatic symptoms, retarded activity and interpersonal difficulties, are the group of symptoms used to diagnose or measure depression[3]. Severity of depression is often determined by a simple sum of depressive symptoms[4,5].

Depressed mood is a single-dimension phenomenon, in lay terms often referred to as feeling depressed or blue. Subsyndromal depression is depressed mood plus at least one other symptom from the standardized list of criteria itemized in the DSM-IV[4]. Minor depressive disorder (mDD) is depressed mood plus two to four other symptoms from the standardized list of criteria, lasting every day for at least two weeks. Major depressive disorder (MDD) is depressed mood (or loss of pleasure) plus at least four other symptoms from the same standardized list, again lasting every day for at least two weeks. These four labels therefore exist on a continuum of increasing numbers of symptoms, with an overlap between subsyndromal and mDD[6]. In addition, specifying the duration of the disorders is required (at least two weeks). The disorders are also defined by an episode based on subsequent relief from the symptoms for another specified duration (in the case of MDD at least two months).

As early as 1976, Craig & Van Natta[7] proposed that duration of symptoms was crucial for diagnosis. The implication that duration of episode is an important part of diagnosis, not necessarily an optional modifier, has been addressed in two diagnoses: recurrent brief depression (RBD) and dysthymia – the former, five criteria from the standardized list lasting less than two weeks and the latter, fewer than five criteria lasting at least two years[8–12]. In summary, RBD, unspecified MDD and MDD with a chronic specifier might be seen as existing on a continuum of increasing duration of episode. Similarly, mDD and dysthymia can be seen as existing on a continuum of increasing duration, although at a lower level of severity than MDD.

Course can be defined as longitudinal pattern of diagnoses, where longitudinal pattern can be seen as a broader term than course, not limited to diagnostic criteria. Heterogeneity in longitudinal pattern has been addressed by requiring or allowing specification in diagnosis of duration of episode, duration of post-episode or interval and frequency of recurrence. Both severity and duration of episode, plus duration of post-episode, and occasionally longitudinal course, have been included – albeit inconsistently – in diagnoses[13,14]. The attempts over the years to differentiate depressions in terms of only some of the dimensions of severity, duration, post-episode duration and course have led to a somewhat inconsistent proliferation of labels and diagnoses.

MENOPAUSE TRANSITION: DEFINITION

Just as there has been lack of clarity in defining depression or depressed mood in studies of depression and menopause, there has also been lack of clarity in definitions of the menopause transition. In Mitchell and colleagues' schema[15], menopausal transition has been divided into three stages: early, middle and late transition (menopausal transition stage, MTS). Women in early transition report changes in either flow or cycle length from age 35 with no changes in cycle regularity. Included in middle transition are those with irregular cycles since age 35 with no skipping of periods. Irregularity was defined as more than six days absolute difference between any two consecutive menstrual cycles during a given year. Late transition includes women who have had one or more episodes of a skipped period. A skipped period was defined as double the modal cycle length or more. In the absence of a modal cycle length, a population-based cycle length of 29 days was used[15]. Most researchers use the terms premenopause and perimenopause, with quite a bit of variability in definitions, although perimenopause often overlaps with late transition at least (see Table 2).

In addition to MTS there are women using hormone therapy and postmenopausal women. The postmenopause group includes women not on hormones who have gone at least 12 months without any bleeding or spotting with no other explanation for their amenorrhea. Women who take hormone therapy (estrogen alone or estrogen with progesterone) would be classified separately from those who are experiencing or have experienced a natural transition to menopause.

NEED FOR LONGITUDINAL STUDIES OF DEPRESSION AND MENOPAUSE

An extensive body of research has investigated depression and menopause[16,17]. Greene[16] reviewed 25 studies and proposed that only those women with the same risk factors for depression at any time of life (low socio-economic status (SES), stressful marriage, unfulfilling employment, bereavement) were vulnerable to depression, and then depression was more likely during the perimenopause than at menopause itself. Nicol-Smith[17] reviewed 94 studies and concluded that the results were not consistent enough to determine a relationship between depression and menopause. In fact, only a few of the studies that were presented graphically demonstrated any relationship, and those few were inconsistent in when or in which stages of menopausal transition or postmenopause there might be a relationship to elevated depressive symptoms. While the author did not critique methods specifically, most of the research has been cross-sectional and often sampled from clinic populations. Research using these methods is still being conducted[18].

As Nicol-Smith reviewed[17], correlation does not imply causality[19,20]. Attempts to link menopause causally to depression would have to consider a temporal relationship, requiring studies with longitudinal design. Nine longitudinal studies of midlife women were identified in the literature, each of which measured depressive symptoms or mental health diagnoses in the same women at more than one time point during the transition to and after menopause. To date, only one longitudinal analysis for each study has been published, with the exception of Bromberger & Matthews[21,22] and Hunter[23,24], who have

Table 1 Longitudinal studies of depression in midlife women

Name of study	Site of study	Senior researcher	Co-authors	Date published
Seattle Midlife Women's Health Study[30]	Seattle, WA	N. F. Woods	Mitchell	1996
University of Pittsburgh Healthy Women Study[21,22]	Allegheny county, PA (includes Pittsburgh)	K. Matthews	Bromberger	1996
Massachusetts Women's Health Study[28]	Massachusetts state	S. McKinlay	Avis, Brambilla, Vass	1994
National Health Examination Follow-up Study[27]	US	P. Costa, Jr.	Busch, Zonderman	1994
Manitoba Project on Women and Their Health in the Middle Years[32]	Manitoba province, Canada	P. Kaufert	Gilbert & Tate	1992
South-East England Study[23,24]	Southeast England, (London and vicinity)	M. Hunter		1990, 1992
Melbourne Women's Midlife Health Project[29]	Melbourne, Australia	L. Dennerstein	Dudley & Burger	1997
Norwegian Menopause Project[26]	Oslo, Norway	A. Holte		1992
Longitudinal Study of Women in Gothenburg[25]	Gothenburg, Sweden	T. Hällström	Samuelsson	1985

published twice. Neither second article had additional information about depressive symptoms and menopausal status. Table 1 provides a summary of study names and researchers. They are arranged in order from smallest to largest geographical area in the US, other English-speaking countries, and lastly other countries.

REVIEW OF THE STUDIES

This review of methodological issues and design focused on sampling methods, size and eligibility criteria, sociocultural characteristics of samples, cohort effects, measurement tools of depression, definitions of menopausal and menstrual status, other independent variables included, study designs and analysis strategies. A summary of these elements from each study has been provided in Tables 2 and 3. Lastly, a review of results in light of methods, design

and analytic strategy completed the purpose of this literature review.

Samples

Sampling methods

Most of the longitudinal studies reviewed here used population- or community-based sampling frames such as tax or community registers[25,26], representative stratified probability sampling[27] or random or stratified sampling of total populations from census list[28], from telephone numbers[29,30], and from drivers' licences[21,22]. Because of the large number of women available in Gothenburg, Hällström and Samuelsson[25] sampled by day of birth within year of birth[31]. All sampling methods of the longitudinal studies produced high participation rates of those contacted and/or eligible for entry to the cross-sectional portions of the studies.

Table 2 Menopausal status in nine longitudinal studies of depressive symptoms in midlife women

Site of study, senior investigator	Menopausal status labels	Number of sub-categories	Definitions
Seattle, Woods (1996)[30]	Not given	Not given	Asked changes in interval and regularity within last 6 months
Allegheny County, PA (including Pittsburgh) Matthews (1996)[21,22]	Premenopausal	3	Menses in last 3 months
	Peri- or postmenopausal		Ceased menses for last 3–12 months
	HRT		Hormone replacement therapy (incl. post-hysterectomy)
Massachusetts, McKinlay (1994)[28]		3	Asked changes within last 9 months
	Premenopausal		Regular menses last 3 months
	Perimenopausal		Periods of amenorrhea and/or changes in regularity or flow past 12 months
	Postmenopause (Natural menopause)		No menses last 12 months
U.S., Costa, Jr. (1994)[27]		4	Based on change from 10 years earlier when regular menses
	Premenopausal		Pregnant or regular menses
	Perimenopausal		Irregular menses due to the change of life
	Natural menopause		No longer menstruating naturally (≥12 months)
	Surgical menopause		No longer menstruating r/t surgery
Manitoba, Kaufert (1992)[32]		4	Asked changes during last 6 months
	Premenopause		Regular menstruation
	Perimenopause		Other than pre, post or hysterectomy
	Postmenopause		No periods × 2 consecutive assessments (= 12 months)
	Hysterectomy		With or without oophorectomy
Melbourne, Dennerstein (1997)[29]	Premenopausal	5	No change in frequency or flow within last 3 months
	Early perimenopausal		Some change in frequency and/or flow within last 3 months
	Late perimenopausal		3–11 months amenorrhea
	Postmenopausal 1		1–2 years amenorrhea
	Postmenopausal 2		>2 years amenorrhea

Continued

Table 2 Continued

Site of study, senior investigator	Menopausal status labels	Number of sub-categories	Definitions
South-East England, Hunter (1990)[23]		3	Change from premenopausal at entry
	Premenopausal	(NB: peri and post combined for analysis)	Regular menses last 12 months
	Perimenopausal		Irregular menses (cycle > 6 weeks)
	Postmenopausal		No menses × 12 or more months
Oslo, Holte (1992)[26]	Premenopause	2	≤ 6 months amenorrhea
	Postmenopause		> 6 months amenorrhea
Gothenburg, Samuelsson (1985)[25]	Preclimacteric	5	38 years old
	Premenopausal		Regular menstruation (no amenorrhea × ≥ 2 months)
	Perimenopausal		Beginning irregular menses (= skipping menses)
	Early postmenopausal		Amenorrhea 12–35 months
	Late postmenopausal		≥ 3 years amenorrhea

Sample sizes

Sample sizes for the longitudinal portions of the studies ranged from a low[23] of 36 to a high[28] of 2352. These sample sizes reflected not only the original geographic areas, ranging from selected census tracts within city limits[30] to the entire US[27], but also the exclusion criteria for the longitudinal portion of studies. The exclusion criteria often eliminated large groups, even the majority, of the original cross-sectional sample[23,26,27,32].

Eligibility criteria

Eligibility criteria for inclusion in the longitudinal analyses varied between the studies reviewed here. Several studies required women be 'premenopausal,' however defined, at entry[21–24,27,32]. For entry to the Massachusetts study women were required to have menstruated within three months; however, they might have been postmenopausal by the time the first measure of depressive symptoms (Center for Epidemiologic Studies Depression Scale, CES-D) was administered, for some women 9 and for some 18 months later[28].

Bromberger and Matthews[21,22] specifically excluded women at entry who were not 'healthy', that is, who were taking anti-depressants and/or other prescription medications or whose depression scores already indicated major depression at entry. They noted that their sample demonstrated a higher SES than non-participants, with higher educational attainment. This finding would be consistent with their requirements for healthy status at entry[33].

Most importantly, several studies specifically excluded women on hormone replacement therapy (HRT) and/or after surgical menopause or hysterectomy[23,25,26,28,29]. Although not explicitly stated, but based on their table of

Table 3 Longitudinal studies of depression during menopausal transition: methods

Site of study (Senior researcher)	Sample size	Sampling method	Calendar years of data collection	Number of time points of measurement	Depression measurement tool	Other independent variables measured	Age at entry to study	Analysis methods
Seattle (Woods)[30]	347	Multistage, community-based telephone numbers	1990–92; 12 months later	2; 1 year apart	CES-D	7 from factor analysis: Social support, Feminine socialization, Health, Vasomotor, Stress, Family Resources, Socialization midlife	35–55	Discriminant analysis; 4-group outcome variable: Absent depressed mood, Consistent depressed mood, Emerging depressed mood, Resolving depressed mood
Allegheny County, PA including Pittsburgh (Matthews)[21,22]	460	Random driver's licenses, selected zip codes; healthy at entry only	1983–85; 1986–88	2; 3 years apart	BDI	History of stressor last 6 months, Current stressor, Pessimism, Trait anxiety, Depression at T1, Education at T1, HRT at T2	42–50	First order correlations; Stepwise linear regression
Massachusetts (McKinlay)[28]	2352 (2347 at end of study)	Random, state census lists	1982–84; 27 months later; through 1987	2; 27 months (2.25 years) apart	CES-D	Hot flashes + night sweats + menstrual problems, HRT at T2, Depression at T1	46–56	Logistic regression; Likelihood ratio test for differences among 5 MTS
US (Costa, Jr.)[27]	394 (sum for CESD calculated, not given)	Stratified probability of adult, non-institutionalized civilian population of U.S.	1971–75; 1982–84	2; 10 years apart	CES-D	Age within menopausal transition stage, Years since menopause	40–58	Repeated measures ANOVA; 2-way MANOVA

Continued

Table 3   Continued

Site of study (P.I.)	Sample size	Sampling method	Calendar years of data collection	Number of time points of measurement	Depression measurement tool	Other independent variables measured	Age at entry to study	Analysis methods
Manitoba, Canada (Kaufert)[32]	469 145 post-hyster-ectomy at entry 324 no hyster-ectomy at entry	Non-random mail survey selected from general population of women in age group in province	1981; 1982; 1983 (est. from publication dates, incl. pilot study)	5 (pooled into 2) 6 months apart	CES-D	Present health Sum of major health problems last 6 months Family events last 6 months: death, children leave Current stress: problems with family, relationships, other	45–55	Chi-square of paired scores from one time point to the next time point (5 time points pooled into multiple pairs) Logistic regression with backward stepwise entry of independent variables
Southeast England (Hunter)[23,24]	36	Volunteer clinical	1983; 1986	2 3 years apart	7-item scale derived from factor analysis of 36 symptom set	Age within menopausal transition stage SES (2 groups) Marital status Employment status Depression at T1 Menopause beliefs Expectations Stress (yes/no) Hypochondriasis Regular exercise	47–55	Paired t-tests and McNemar tests Multiple stepwise regression
Melbourne, Australia (Dennerstein)[29]	438 (405 at end of year 4)	Random, community-based, Australian-born	1991; 1992; 1993; 1994	4 (pooled) 1 year apart	Affectometer 2	Age adjusted for menopausal trans stage Free estradiol Estradiol index Free FSH Free androgen index Hot flashes (bother-some, last 2 weeks)	45–55	Generalized linear model, pooled data set assuming normal errors, stepwise entry of variables

Continued

Table 3 Continued

Site of study (P.I.)	Sample size	Sampling method	Calendar years of data collection	Number of time points of measurement	Depression measurement tool	Other independent variables measured	Age at entry to study	Analysis methods
Oslo, Norway (Holte)[26]	59	Random, Community Register of Central Bureau of Statistics	1981; 1982; 1983; 1984; 1985; 1986	5⇒2 dichotomized to pre and post menopause 1 year apart	4-item yes/no scale from GHQ + 3 questions for each item: 1. Current yes/no 2. Frequency in last 12 months (12-pt) 3. Amount of distress (4-pt)	Age Age within menopausal transition stage Vasomotor sx	47–56	t-test of summary measures pre vs post menopause
Gothenberg, Sweden (Hällström)[25]	677	Systematic, Taxation Office Register	1968–69; 1974–75	2 6 years apart	DSM-III criteria, semi-structured psychiatric interview	Age at entry Marital status No. of children Social class Employment (0,PT,FT) Weighted life events (complex measure)	38–54	Nonparametric comparisons (Pitman's permutation test, Fisher's permutation test, or Fisher's exact test) of percentages or rates, with Mantel method of adjustment for confounding variables

CES-D, Center for Epidemiologic Studies Depression Scale; BDI, Beck Depression Inventory; HRT, hormone replacement therapy; MTS, menopausal transition stage; SES, socio-economic status; FSH, follicle-stimulating hormone; GHQ, General Health Questionnaire; DSM-III, Diagnostic and Statistical Manual, 3rd edn.

sample characteristics, Avis and colleagues[28] apparently excluded women on HRT at entry to the longitudinal study, but retained them in the sample if later they had used HRT. Rates of HRT use were therefore very low in their sample: 5.1% among women who had not had hysterectomies.

Yet, if the purpose of the study was to investigate the effect of menopausal or menstrual status or its change on depressive symptoms, eliminating portions of the sample due to use of HRT, for example, meant that the researcher lost one of the common intervening variables possibly related to depression, if the depressive symptoms were the reason why the women received HRT and/or hysterectomy. It is well-established that many women with depression somatize and present with gynecologic complaints[34], the latter often leading to HRT prescription and/or hysterectomy in midlife[35]. It is also common practice for midlife women with depressive symptoms to be prescribed HRT[36–39]. Therefore, excluding those women from the sample created a bias in determining the relationship between menopausal status and depression.

In fact, the reason these nine studies were conducted was due to the common professional and popular belief that menopausal transition causes depression. Based on this belief, the logical intervention is to treat the depression by treating the menopausal transition, namely by prescribing HRT. However, this practice means that studies excluding women on HRT might have, in essence, excluded the portion of their outcome variable that they were most interested in. Elimination of HRT users was particularly problematic when this group comprised a large minority of the original cross-sectional sample[26]. Caution is warranted therefore in comparing results between studies and especially in generalizing them to all midlife women.

Sociocultural characteristics of samples

Sociocultural differences between countries and even between regions within the US might

also have contributed to differences in outcomes. While the focus of the present research was not cross-cultural, many other investigators have studied such differences[40–47]. The nine longitudinal studies reviewed here compared in their discussions women living in Sweden, Norway, Australia, England, Canada and various regions of and the whole of the US. Assumptions of cross-country similarities were not made explicit but implied by Hunter[48] in discussing five of the longitudinal studies also reviewed here, that women in all five countries were readily comparable.

Cohort effects

Cohort effects refer to bias or confounding based on historical changes in factors influencing the outcome variable[49]. For example, women born earlier last century were less likely to have had paid employment than women born more recently. If paid employment affected depressive symptoms, then women might be expected to have varying rates of depressive symptoms due to differences in employment history between age groups (cohorts)[50]. In this review, cohort effects would have been determined by the year in which the data were collected combined with the age of the women in that year. The earliest data collection occurred in 1968 in a Gothenburg study with women as old as 54 years[25] while the latest occurred in Melbourne in 1994 with women as young as 49 years[29] and in Seattle in 1991 with women as young as 35 years[30].

Measurement tools

All of the researchers used self-reported symptom measures of depression except Hällström and Samuelsson[25] in Gothenburg, Sweden. Some of the self-reports were done by mail questionnaire, some by telephone or personal interview. The most frequently used tool (see Table 3) was the Center for Epidemiologic Studies Depression (CES-D) Scale[3]. Other tools included standardized ones such as the Beck Depression Inventory (BDI), used in Pittsburgh[21,22], an adaptation of the General

Health Questionnaire (GHQ) used in Norway[26], and an adaptation of the Affectometer-2 used in Melbourne[29]. Through principal components analysis Hunter developed a measure of depression from a set of 36 symptoms from the Women's Health Questionnaire[22,23].

Self-report measures of depressive symptoms were developed for ease of administration in research studies and were "designed to measure current level of depressive symptomatology, with emphasis on the affective component [and] depressed mood" (Radloff, 1977)[3]. Hällström and Samuelsson, in Gothenburg[25], were the only researchers to conduct psychiatric interviews to establish actual diagnoses of mental health problems. They used a semi-structured interview that lasted from one-half to two hours[31]. Unfortunately, a potential bias was introduced by their procedure of one researcher (Hällström) conducting all of the interviews for the first wave and the other (Samuelsson) conducting all of the interviews for the second wave. Their inter-rater reliabilities were generally high, but in the one area of psychiatrist-observed behavior, inter-rater reliabilities were so low as to be unusable[31].

Measurement of menopausal and menstrual status

While the variable of menopausal/menstrual status was only one of several that were included in the nine studies, it was isolated for review here because of its central importance for longitudinal studies of menopause and depression (see Table 2). Conceptual issues in defining menopausal status were reviewed in 1987 by Kaufert and colleagues[51]. As they pointed out, commonly used categories of menopausal status were derived from only a limited amount of empirical information, particularly scant hormonal information but also little cycle and flow data as well. For example, in their own longitudinal analysis, Kaufert and associates[51] started with, but provided no particular basis for, a menopausal status of amenorrhea for three months and in fact ended up combining this category with

irregular cycles. In addition, according to their own data (and replicated in Holte's study[26]) amenorrhea for six months, initially a separate category, was actually the beginning of postmenopause in over 90% of women, who continued on to 12 months of amenorrhea. Their purpose in combining irregular menstruation with amenorrhea for the previous three months was "to simplify presentation"[51]. Their purpose in separating the category of 'amenorrhea for the last three months' from 'amenorrhea for the last six months' was not provided. The limited empirical basis for definitions of menopausal status creates the potential for uncertainty in classification, as evidenced by the Manitoba researchers, and even misclassification.

Designs

All of the studies reviewed here were prospective and observational in design. Longitudinal research designs must also specify the number and timing of data collection points (see Table 3). Three of the nine longitudinal studies measured depressive symptoms more than two times: Kaufert and co-workers[32] measured six although they had to discard the final one in analysis because of problems with implementation. Dennerstein and colleagues[29] measured four, and Holte[26] measured six although the latter aggregated results into two summary measures. None of these were US studies.

Timing of the data collection ranged from six months apart in Manitoba to ten years apart for the National Health Examination Follow-up Study (NHEFS), with three studies using a time interval of one year. While Avis and colleagues[28] contacted Massachusetts women every nine months, the CES-D was administered at only two time points 27 months apart. Those studies that used the most number of measurement occasions also used the shortest time intervals (see Table 3).

No researcher provided a rationale for the time interval either in terms of theory or existing research regarding changes in depressive symptoms or changes in menopausal/menstrual status. Research on MDD has indicated that several months are required for intervention to have effect for those women that are diagnosed, treated and respond[52-59]. Therefore, measuring CES-D scores every six months, as the Manitoba researchers did, would be very likely to capture change from an episode to remission or recovery, and measurement every nine or even 12 months, as the Massachusetts, Seattle, Melbourne and Norwegian researchers did, would also be likely to identify changes in depressive symptoms. Longer time intervals between measurements could possibly miss depressive episodes and/or recoveries. As for MTS, middle and late transition combined have been determined to last approximately six years on average (Ellen S. Mitchell, personal communication). Thus, depressive symptoms would have to be measured over several years in order to allow enough of the women being followed to change at least once from one MTS to another for true longitudinal design.

Measurement of MTS also relates to research design. Most of the researchers reviewed here seemed to assume that a particular status, that is, being perimenopausal or being postmenopausal (however defined, see Table 2) might relate significantly to depressive symptoms. However, as Kaufert and associates pointed out[51]: "researchers cannot discriminate between women close to a change in their menopausal status and those whose status will remain relatively stable for a year or more". One reason researchers cannot discriminate is that the changes of menopausal transition do not necessarily occur in a forward linear progression. In addition, as Mitchell and colleagues have described[15], each stage of the transition lasts on average two or three years; however, an individual woman might experience a shorter or longer stage than the average. Thus for the researcher, the first months of perimenopause, or late transition for example, will be classified similarly to the last months, the latter perhaps being three years later, at the final menstrual period itself.

Avis and colleagues[28], Kaufert and co-workers[32] and Busch *et al*[27] used change in status as the factor that might be related to depressive symptoms. For the latter group, the

three categories were women who (after being selected as premenopausal at time one) had stayed premenopausal, had become perimenopausal, or had become postmenopausal at time two. The former groups used similar time-paired status categories. Avis and colleagues[28] found another aspect of status – the duration of time within perimenopause – significant. It might be important for future researchers to be able to consider all three aspects of menopausal status: being in a stage, changing from or to a stage, and duration of time in a particular stage of the menopausal transition.

Results

Given the difficulties already reviewed in comparing these nine longitudinal studies of depression during the menopausal transition, the general consistency of negative results is all the more remarkable. Five of the studies reviewed here found no relationship between menopausal status or a change in menopausal status and depressive symptoms. All of the studies that were designed for it found that the single best predictor of depression at a later time point was depression at an earlier time point, unrelated to menopausal status or its change. Three studies found significant relationships between depressive symptoms and menopausal status: South-East England, the only study to use clinical sampling (Hunter[23,24]); Massachusetts (Avis and co-workers[28]); and Melbourne (Dennerstein and colleagues[29]). First, each study's results have been summarized for the relationship between depression and menopausal status. Secondly, effects of covariates or predictors are reviewed. Lastly, comparisons to other studies have been included where meaningful.

Seattle Midlife Women's Health Study

Woods and Mitchell[30] did not find menstrual changes to significantly predict depressive symptoms or their pattern of change. However, the Seattle researchers did find different variable groups from a factor analysis to discriminate between change patterns, including previous history of depression such as premenstrual syndrome or postpartum depression, stress, health status, socialization, family resources and social support. The pattern of consistent depressed mood was discriminated from the pattern of resolving depressed mood additionally by vasomotor symptoms. The predictors could be interpreted as history of previous depression and life events and stressors, allowing for a buffering effect of resources and support. As an additional note about pattern, while these authors did not provide the results in this form, 22% of women changed category of depressive symptoms in one year, 41 of 347 increasing their scores to over the CES-D cutoff of ≥ 16, and 36 of 347 decreasing below it. Thus, 78% of the women were stable over the one year interval.

University Of Pittsburgh Healthy Women Study

Bromberger and Matthews[21,22] found that neither HRT use compared to premenopausal status, nor combined peri- and postmenopausal status compared to premenopausal status, contributed significantly to the outcome of depressive symptoms. They also examined individual correlations between each individual measure and depressive symptoms at follow-up and found that depressive symptom score at entry had the highest, and a statistically significant, correlation. Depressive symptom score at Time 1 was also the significant predictor of highest magnitude in a multiple regression model for prediction of Time 2 depressive symptoms. Measures of trait anxiety, stress as an ongoing problem and stress as a recent event were also significant predictors at lesser magnitudes. Thus, life events and stressors were also predictive of midlife depressive symptoms.

Massachusetts Women's Health Study

Of the three studies where significant differences were obtained in depressive symptoms by menopausal status, the Massachusetts study[28] was the one with the largest sample size. They found significantly higher depression scores in the group of women who were perimenopausal at both time points, 27 months (2.25 years) apart. This higher rate of depressive symptoms was found when compared with women who were premenopausal at both time points, women who were postmenopausal at both time points and women who had changed status. The measure of significance was not dramatic, with the p value given as < 0.05 and the lower limit of the 95% confidence interval of the odds ratio given as 1.05; a confidence interval including 1 would not have been significant. The significant difference between the group of women perimenopausal at both time points and other groups was not maintained when the logistic regression model was adjusted for menstrual problems. The significant results of the Massachusetts study can be evaluated in terms of the sample size, the definition of menstrual problems, and the definitions of pre- and perimenopause.

The Massachusetts study had by far the largest sample of the nine studies reviewed in this chapter, which makes their results noteworthy but also enhanced their chances of finding statistical significance for small differences. Hot flashes, night sweats, and "menstrual problems" were combined into a single predictor variable in their logistic regression model. The reason these variables were combined was because "none of the women in the pre/peri-post and post-post groups reported menstrual problems"; however, "menstrual problems" (Magursky and colleagues[60]) were understood to be the defining criteria of early and middle transition. It was therefore not surprising that it was mostly the peri-peri group that complained of these 'problems'. When the model was adjusted for menstrual problems alone without vasomotor symptoms, there were still no differences in depression scores between MTS groups.

In their discussion, Avis and colleagues[28] acknowledged that menopausal symptoms might be an expression of depression; in that case they would have adjusted for a dimension of their outcome variable itself, an adjustment that did indeed result in loss of significance between MTS groups. In other analyses the Massachusetts researchers noted that women who had psychological complaints also tended to have complaints about all symptoms[61] and to have had most of the same complaints prior to menopausal transition[62]. Women were excluded in the longitudinal analysis who had hysterectomies by the second time point, a group that had the highest CES-D scores in their cross-sectional analysis[62].

Definitions of perimenopause and prolonged perimenopause might have been problematic; their definitions of MTS were not mutually exclusive. Women could have experienced three months of regular periods immediately before the interview, to be classified as premenopausal, and still have experienced periods of amenorrhea and/or changes in regularity or flow during the previous 12 months, classified as perimenopausal. Since women who were complaining of menstrual problems – that is, complaining of the characteristics that define middle and late transition – were also the same women who tended to complain about all symptoms, including depressive ones, it was possible that women who were classified as perimenopausal, especially at both time points, were those women who were more likely to have depressive symptoms. This misclassification bias would explain the significant results of prolonged perimenopause being a predictor of high CES-D score.

Avis and colleagues[28] described their results as a transitory increase in depressive symptoms during the perimenopause. In actuality, however, it was not known if the persistently perimenopausal women had low depression scores before perimenopause and/or would have low scores when postmenopausal. A transitory increase does not explain why women who were perimenopausal at the second time point only – premenopausal becoming perimenopausal – did not show a significant difference from the reference group of women premenopausal at both time points. Their ability to determine whether depression scores decreased after perimenopause was also limited by not using a change category of peri becoming post. Instead, they

combined pre- and perimenopause into one for a change category of pre/peri becoming post. Similar to the University of Pittsburgh, Manitoba (see later), and Seattle studies and an earlier cross-sectional analysis[62], their longitudinal analysis found a previous history of depressive symptoms to be the strongest predictor of perimenopausal depressive symptoms.

Because of the differences in designs and analyses between the Massachusetts study and the other studies reviewed here, however, neither refutation nor replication of the Massachusetts results was possible. The University of Pittsburgh study combined peri- and postmenopausal women into one category and thus by design could not have determined an effect of any form of perimenopause alone, prolonged or otherwise – only the effect of change to not having menstrual periods within at least the previous three months. The South-East England study admitted women to the longitudinal study only if they were premenopausal at the first time point and then combined peri- with postmenopause; similar to the University of Pittsburgh study, by design the South-East England study could not have determined effects of any form of perimenopause, prolonged or otherwise.

Woods and Mitchell[30] did not include a long enough time span, only 12 months apart, to be able to replicate the prolonged perimenopause of the Massachusetts study. Also, the majority of the Seattle women were in early or middle transition, not late transition when MTS changes would have been most similar to 'prolonged perimenopause'. The NHEFS and Gothenburg studies measured depression at time points too far apart, ten years and six years respectively, to replicate any effects of 'prolonged perimenopause'. The NHEFS pointed out themselves that significant increases in depression scores might have occurred and resolved within the ten years between their two data collection points. Also, by design, all women in the NHEFS were premenopausal at time one, so for that reason, too, they could not replicate the findings for prolonged perimenopause of the Massachusetts study. Again by design, Holte did not include perimenopause as a variable and thus could not have determined any effect it might have had on depressive symptoms[26].

The Manitoba study[32] analyzed change only between time points six months apart and could not have replicated any effects of prolonged perimenopause either. However, it was possible that if Kaufert and colleagues had examined data for women who remained perimenopausal across 27 months or longer and then compared them to other women they might have replicated McKinlay's findings. The Melbourne study analyzed each data point as if independent, so they, too, could not have found any effects of 'prolonged perimenopause'.

National Health Examination Follow-up Study

Busch and colleagues[27] found no effect of MTS change group on depressive symptoms, and otherwise measured only age within MTS. They included a caution that in their study "subjects exceeding the cutoff point for depression [at Time 1] were less likely to be traced [for Time 2 follow-up] than were non-depressed subjects", possibly affecting the negative results through selection bias. Because of the ten-year time interval, the lack of covariates or predictors, and the recognized bias in the follow-up sample, it was difficult to compare these results to those of other studies.

Manitoba Project On Women And Their Health In The Middle Years

The Manitoba study[32] found no relationship between change in depression score and menopausal status or change in menopausal status and depression score. Starting with χ^2 analyses these researchers did find significantly increased likelihood of depression scores at 'time two' (see later in this subsection) in those women with hysterectomy at any point who had not been depressed at 'time one', compared to all other women. The relative odds of depression at time two in this group were 1.7 (95% C.I. 1.15–2.6).

The multiple logistic regression models with backward stepwise entry of variables con-

firmed the results of the series of χ^2 analyses where "menopausal status categories were entered as dummy variables". After adjustment for other independent variables predictors of higher depressive symptoms at time two after lower depressive symptoms at time one included poor self-rating of health status, diagnoses of arthritis or high blood pressure or self-rating of problems with husband, children, other relationships or other areas of life. Variables predictive of staying depressed at time two after being depressed at time one again included a poor self-rating of health status and diagnoses of three or more other health problems. Confusingly, diagnosis of arthritis or thyroid problems was reported in the narrative results as significantly associated with staying depressed; however, significance levels were reported as 0.08 and 0.04, respectively, but the confidence intervals reported for both of these odds ratios included 1.

Understanding the effects of hysterectomy was also problematic. Because of the technique of pooling or collapsing the five longitudinal data measurements into pairs of time points, 'time one' might have been any one of the measurements one to four; 'time two' might have been any one of the measurements two to five. Hysterectomy might not have occurred during the particular six-month interval between 'time one' and 'time two' when rise in depression score occurred. Yet if hysterectomy had occurred at any time during the study, the woman was more likely to have a pair of six month depression scores where score at 'time two' was high after a high 'time one' score. Generally, the analytic technique of pooling made significant results uninterpretable. Another possible explanation for the Manitoba study's results was a Type I error resulting from "a series of" χ^2 analyses performed without accommodation for multiple comparisons, i.e. this one significant result was due to chance.

Comparison of these significant results with other studies were not possible because most of the studies excluded women who had hysterectomies; only the Massachusetts, NHEFS and University of Pittsburgh studies included women who had hysterectomies, and the University of Pittsburgh study included them in the HRT group in general. These other studies found no evidence of increased depression scores in the HRT/hysterectomy group. Thus, of the four studies that included women with hysterectomies, only the 1992 Manitoba study[32] found hysterectomy to be predictive for increase in depression scores, and then only in the subgroup who were not consistently depressed. Of the other three studies that found significant increase in depressive symptoms with some stage of MTS[23,24,28], none included women who had hysterectomies.

Another set of results from the Manitoba study was unique, however. This study was the only one, other than a few case examples in the Norwegian article[26], that presented results of longitudinally repeated measures, although no statistical analyses were performed. While Kaufert and co-workers[32] might be critiqued for analytic strategies that failed to account for inter-individual correlation of repeated measures, this presentation avoided that criticism. They displayed patterns over time of CES-D scores along with the number of women demonstrating each pattern. The CES-D score was classified as dichotomous, ≥ 16 and < 16 in black and white boxes, respectively. Even with some patterns not present, they observed 29 out of a possible total of 32 or 2^5 patterns. While numbers of women demonstrating each longitudinal pattern were provided, little interpretation or discussion was added. In their earlier article using the same format for presentation of longitudinal patterns of menstrual changes, they wrote that "this manner of presentation is too detailed for interpretation"[51].

South-East England Study

Hunter[23,24] was the only researcher who found in both cross-sectional[64] and longitudinal analyses that the group of combined peri- and postmenopausal women experienced increased depressive symptoms over premenopausal women. These results might have been due to the combining of and/or definitions of MTS, cultural differences of women in South-East

England, the small sample size (36 total), the use of clinical sampling, or chance results. The use of the clinical sample was the most likely reason for the significance of the results[65]. Bromberger and Matthews[21,22] also combined peri- and postmenopause and compared depressive symptoms to premenopause but found no significant differences. Results of the South-East England Study were not comparable to other studies because of the sampling methods and definitions used of MTS.

Melbourne Women's Midlife Health Project

Dennerstein and colleagues found significant differences in depressive symptoms comparing pre- to perimenopause and comparing pre- to early postmenopause only in their longitudinal analysis[29], not in their cross-sectional analysis[66]. In the longitudinal study, negative affect in late postmenopause also was not significantly different from premenopause. Higher negative affect for peri- and early postmenopause remained significant even after hot flashes were included in the regression model, although this finding was not true for a measure of positive affect. None of the hormonal assays of estradiol (E_2), free androgen index (FAI), follicle stimulating hormone (FSH) or serum hormone binding globulin (SHBG), or hot flashes, contributed significantly to the model of CES-D score after MTS was already entered. Since hormonal assays and MTS had been found to be correlated, this result was not surprising.

Similar to Avis and colleagues' study[28], the Melbourne study described the increase in negative affect as temporary because of the lack of significant difference between pre- and late postmenopause. However, in the Melbourne study, changes in depression scores across time for an individual woman could not be determined because of their analysis strategy of treating each longitudinal data point as independent, thus analyzing their longitudinal data set as if cross-sectional.

By their own admission this analysis did not include the variables of health status, stress, marital status, premenstrual complaints and lifestyle that these same researchers found "significantly related" to well-being[29] in their cross-sectional analyses[66,67]. In light of the inter-individual correlations in the 'pooled' longitudinal data set and the omission of previously significant predictors in the model, a finding of statistical significance was uninterpretable.

Norwegian Menopause Project

The only study using multiple time points and an appropriate analytic strategy, by Holte[26] in 1992, did not find any relationship between the menopause and depressive symptoms; a mean premenopause score was compared by paired t-test to a mean postmenopause score. Social dysfunction, a possible indicator of depression, was significantly related to vasomotor complaints. Difficulties in comparing this study with others was based on the analytic strategy and design.

Longitudinal Study Of Women In Gothenburg

The Gothenburg researchers, Hällström and Samuelsson[25], were the only ones to diagnose depressive disorder, although only as one category of mental health problems albeit the majority of them. They also measured level of disability from mental health problems. They found no relationship between mental health problems or disability and MTS. These researchers also found, by retrospective recall, that the best predictor of a major depressive episode in midlife was a history of earlier depressive symptoms. The Gothenburg study also investigated onset rate or incidence of mental disorders, using recall for the previous year, and found that rates were constant throughout the menopausal transition, and also unrelated to MTS. The implications of this finding were that some women did experience a first major depressive episode during midlife, but the rates for first episode were not increased because of menopausal transition. Women who were divorced, childless and of lower SES had higher prevalences and incidences of mental disorder than women of higher SES who were married with children. These predictors could be interpreted as life events and stressors.

While not statistically significant, a trend toward a cohort effect was evident. Women who were in the oldest age group at entry had higher prevalences of mental disorders at both measurement points than younger women at either measurement point. However, there was no trend for increasing prevalence within any age cohort from first to second measurement point, regardless of MTS. Because the Gothenburg study was the earliest longitudinal research on depressive symptoms and menopausal transition (first wave in 1968), its findings of no relationship between these two phenomena were reassuring about the lack of cohort effects.

Summary

In summary, few longitudinal studies of depression or depressive symptoms in midlife women have found an increase in depression, and those few used clinical sampling[23,24], or statistical methods whose assumptions were not met[29,32], or definitions of MTS that were not mutually exclusive and might have biased inclusion of women with higher depressive symptoms into the perimenopause category[28]. In other words, the longitudinal studies of depression during the menopausal transition that found an increase in or higher depression during perimenopause had methodological flaws to which the differences can be attributed. The majority of longitudinal studies found no relationship between depressive symptoms and menopausal transition or menopause.

Those studies that were able to include it in their models or analysis strategies found that the single best predictor of depressive symptoms at the second time point was level of depressive symptoms at the first. This finding was consistent with those of the course of depression; it would be expected that by midlife a majority of depressive episodes would be recurrences or relapses, perhaps not any more likely to be related to menopausal transition than recurrences or relapses at other ages would be related to menses[68].

Those studies that were designed to include a measure of life events or stressors[21–25,30,32] found significant relationships between some measure of life events and/or stressors, although Bromberger and Matthews[21,22] found significance only in an interaction with anxiety and Hunter[23] only when previous depressive symptoms were removed from the multiple regression model.

General criticisms of the nine studies reviewed here included sampling frames and methods that limited external validity (South-East England); sample sizes that were too small to establish reliability of estimates (South-East England, Norway); a general assumption of comparability across different countries; lack of consistency in definition of an important independent variable, MTS; and, except for three studies, measurement at only two time points. Often, studies excluded an important segment of the sample related to the outcome variable; several excluded HRT users, women with surgical menopause, or, as the Norwegian study did, excluded women in what might have been "prolonged perimenopause".

Six of the studies were limited to only two time points – in one study[30] very close together (one year) and in another[27] very far apart (10 years). Only one of the three studies with multiple time points of measurement used an analytic technique that accounted for inter-individual correlation[26], and that study aggregated observations into two summary measures for a simple comparison pre and post final menstrual period, thereby losing some longitudinal information about patterns. Two of the three studies with multiple time points[29,32] used analyses with 'pooling' of intra-individually repeated measures as if they were independent observations.

Each of the studies reviewed have contributed to understanding changes in depressive symptoms during the menopausal transition and how best to study them. Woods and Mitchell[30] investigated the rich context of women's lives, including resources and support, for analysis of depressive symptoms; they also investigated change in depressive symptoms and menopausal/menstrual status during midlife. Avis and colleagues[28] utilized the largest sample size, thus providing the most reliable estimates of effects, and included

a measure of change. Bromberger and Matthews[21,22] included consideration of psychological theories of depression, in particular theories relating depression to personality, and included a measure of change. Busch and co-workers[27] included the epidemiologically important categories of surgical menopause and HRT use, included a measure of change, and used an age variable adjusted for MTS. Kaufert and colleagues[32] were the only researchers to present multi-point longitudinal patterns of depression scores, and they used the shortest time interval between data collections as well. In addition, they included epidemiologically important categories of surgical menopause and HRT users. They also measured change. Dennerstein and colleagues[29] were one of the few research teams to emphasize wellness and well-being, not just illness and disease. To date they are also the only researchers of longitudinal depressive symptoms in midlife to report assessment of hormonal levels as well as MTS. Hunter[23,24] used a psychological theory of depression to investigate predictors and covariates in depth. Holte[26] was the single researcher to use multi-point data collection and an analytic technique that accommodated intra-individual correlation of repeated measures. The Gothenberg study[25] was able to determine psychiatric diagnoses by expert interview, included all mental health disorders and associated levels of disability, and determined incidence rates during midlife. The latter were particularly important in terms of longitudinal patterns of depressive symptoms during midlife.

No single study of longitudinal depression during the transition to menopause has been without both strengths and weaknesses. The study that remains to be done would combine strengths from the examples reviewed here while avoiding their weaknesses. This study's characteristics would be: (1) adequately-sized population-based sampling; (2) measurement of covariates and predictors related to depression, such as history of depression, use of therapies for depressive symptoms, life events and stressors, including history of violence; (3) use of evidence-based definitions of MTS applied to prospectively collected data; (4) measurement at multiple time points spaced both closely enough and over a long enough time period to capture change in both depressive symptoms and MTS; and (5) use of appropriate analytic strategies for repeated measures.

SIGNIFICANCE

If both course and causes, or at least predictors, of depression were better understood, midlife women who were depressed might be provided with more appropriate therapies and interventions. In particular, if aspects of the menopausal transition and/or menopause are causal or contribute to depressive symptoms in midlife, primary prevention, targeted screening and early diagnosis – and especially efforts to shorten the course of and prevent recurrences of depression – might be more effectively designed. For example, HRT or ERT have become popular approaches to treatment of depressive symptoms in midlife women[69,70]. So far as psychosocial aspects of menopause are concerned, various 'beauty' products are vigorously marketed to prevent the appearance of aging in women[2], a worry that might lead to depression. Increased social activities or employment have been proposed for empty nest syndrome[2,71].

However, if depressive symptoms in midlife are not related to the menopausal transition and menopause, a different focus might be adopted – a focus on depressive symptoms rather than on menopause. If, for example, depressive symptoms are related to life events and stressors, then understanding the relationships between them would be helpful in designing interventions. If depressive symptoms in midlife women are related to previous depressive symptoms, then an understanding of the longitudinal pattern of depressive symptoms would be necessary to predict and hopefully intervene effectively during this time of life for women.

The Seattle Midlife Women's Health Study[29] (SMWHS) can fill many gaps and avoid many pitfalls in the research literature on longitudinal depressive symptoms during the menopausal transition. SMWHS measured depressive symptoms both frequently enough (every year) and for a long enough time period (up to ten years) for changes in both MTS and depressive symptoms to be determined. Measurements of possible causal factors were also available and most data had been recorded prospectively. The sample was from the Seattle community, not clinical practices or diagnosed patients, and was fairly large: over 200 women providing the multi-time-point data. MTS had been determined prospectively and precisely for the participants. Women who had hysterectomy without bilateral oophorectomy or who used HRT were included. Analytic methods could be applied that capitalized on the multi-time-point data set while not violating statistical assumptions. These factors provided an excellent opportunity to explore and describe longitudinal patterns of depressive symptoms in a community-based sample of midlife women during the menopausal transition.

References

1. Woods NF, Mitchell ES. Anticipating menopause: observations from the Seattle Midlife Women's Health Study. *Menopause* 1999;6: 167–73
2. Stoppard JM. *Understanding Depression: Feminist Social Constructionist Approaches*. London and New York: Routledge, 2000
3. Radloff LS. The CES-D Scale: a self-report depression scale for research in the general population. *Appl Psychol Measurement* 1977;1: 385–401
4. American Psychiatric Association Committee on Nomenclature and Statistics. Mood disorders. In *Diagnostic and Statistical Manual of Mental Disorders (DSM-IV)*, 4th edn. Washington: American Psychiatric Association, 1994:317–91
5. Chen L, Eaton WW, Gallo JJ, *et al.* Understanding the heterogeneity of depression through the triad of symptoms, course and risk factors: a longitudinal, population-based study. *J Affect Disord* 2000;59:1–11
6. Judd LL. Pleomorphic expressions of unipolar

depressive disease: summary of the 1996 CINP President's Workshop. *J Affect Disord* 1997;45: 109–16

7. Craig TJ, Van Natta PA. Presence and persistence of depressive symptoms in patient and community populations. *Am J Psychiatry* 1976; 133:1426–9

8. Angst J, Hochstrasser B. Recurrent brief depression: the Zurich study. *J Clin Psychiatry* 1994;55 suppl:3–9

9. Lepine J-P, Pelissolo A, Weiller E, *et al.* Recurrent brief depression: clinical and epidemiological issues. *Psychopathology* 1995;28 Suppl 1:86–94

10. Keller MB, Hanks DL, Klein DN. Summary of the DSM-IV mood disorders field trial and issue overview. *Psychiatr Clin North Am* 1996;19:1–28

11. Keller MB, Hirschfeld RMA, Hanks D. Double depression: a distinctive subtype of unipolar depression. *J Affect Disord* 1997;45:65–73

12. Klein DN, Kocsis JH, McCullough JP, *et al.* Symptomatology in dysthymic and major depressive disorder. *Psychiatr Clin North Am* 1996;19:41–53

13. First MB, Donovan S, Frances A. Nosology of chronic mood disorders. *Psychiatr Clin North Am* 1996;19:29–39

14. McCullough JP, Kornstein SG, McCullough JP, *et al.* Differential diagnosis of chronic depressive disorders. *Psychiatr Clin North Am* 1996;19: 55–71

15. Mitchell ES, Woods NF, Mariella A. Three stages of the menopausal transition from the Seattle Midlife Women's Health Study: toward a more precise definition. *Menopause* 2000;7:334–49

16. Greene JG. The cross-sectional legacy: an introduction to longitudinal studies of the climacteric. *Maturitas* 1992;14:95–101

17. Nicol-Smith L. Causality, menopause and depression: a critical review of the literature. *BMJ* 1996;313:1229–32

18. Sagsoz N, Oguzturk O, Bayram M, *et al.* Anxiety and depression before and after the menopause (abstract). *Arch Gynecol Obstet* 2001;264: 199–202

19. Kleinbaum DG, Kupper LL, Muller KE. *Applied Regression Analysis and other Multivariable Methods*, 2nd edn. Boston: PWS-Kent Publishing, 1988

20. Rothman KJ. *Modern Epidemiology*. Boston: Little, Brown, 1986

21. Bromberger JT, Matthews KA. A "feminine" model of vulnerability to depressive symptoms: a longitudinal investigation of middle-aged women. *J Pers Soc Psychol* 1996;70:591–8

22. Bromberger JT, Matthews KA. A longitudinal study of the effects of pessimism, trait anxiety, and life stress on depressive symptoms in middle-aged women. *Psychol Aging* 1996;11: 207–13

23. Hunter MS. Somatic experience of the menopause: a prospective study. *Psychosom Med* 1990; 52:357–67

24. Hunter M. The Southeast England longitudinal study of the climacteric and postmenopause. *Maturitas* 1992;14:117–26

25. Hällström T, Samuelsson S. Mental health in the climacteric: the longitudinal study of women in Gothenburg. *Acta Obstet Gynecol Scand Suppl* 1985;130:13–18

26. Holte A. Influences of natural menopause on health complaints: a prospective study of healthy Norwegian women. *Maturitas* 1992;14: 127–41

27. Busch CM, Zonderman AB, Costa Jr. PT. Menopausal transition and psychological distress in a nationally representative sample: is menopause associated with psychological distress? *J Aging Health* 1994;6:209–28

28. Avis NE, Brambilla D, McKinlay SM, *et al.* A longitudinal analysis of the association between menopause and depression: results from the Massachusetts Women's Health Study. *Ann Epidemiol* 1994;4:214–20

29. Dennerstein L, Dudley E, Burger H. Well-being and the menopausal transition. *J Psychosom Obstet Gynecol* 1997;18:95–101

30. Woods NF, Mitchell ES. Patterns of depressed mood in midlife women: observations from the Seattle Midlife Women's Health Study. *Res Nurs Health* 1996;19:111–23

31. Samuelsson S. Life events and mental disorder in an urban female population. *Acta Psychiatr Scand Suppl* 1982;299:1–76

32. Kaufert PA, Gilbert P, Tate R. The Manitoba Project: a re-examination of the link between menopause and depression. *Maturitas* 1992;14: 143–55

33. Haan M, Kaplan GA, Camacho T. Poverty and health: prospective evidence from the Alameda County study. *Am J Epidemiol* 1987;125:989–98

34. Kirmayer LJ, Robbins JM. Patients who somatize in primary care: a longitudinal study of cognitive and social characteristics. *Psychol Med* 1996;26:937–51

35. Gath D, Cooper P, Day A. Hysterectomy and psychiatric disorder: I. Levels of psychiatric morbidity before and after hysterectomy. *Br J Psychiatry* 1982;140:335–42

36. Derby CA, Hume AL, Barbour MM, *et al.* Correlates of postmenopausal estrogen use and trends through the 1980s in two southeastern New England communities. *Am J Epidemiol* 1993;137:1125–35

37. Hemminki E, Kennedy DL, Baum C, *et al.* Prescribing of noncontraceptive estrogens and progestins in the United States, 1974–86. *Am J Public Health* 1988;78:1479–81

38. Klaiber EL, Broverman DM, Vogel W, *et al.*

Estrogen therapy for severe persistent depressions in women. *Arch Gen Psychiatry* 1979;36: 550–4

39. Strickler RC, Borth R, Cecutti A, *et al.* The role of oestrogen replacement in the climacteric syndrome. *Psychol Med* 1977;7:631–9

40. Beyene Y. Cultural significance and physiological manifestations of menopause: a biocultural analysis. *Cult Med Psychiatry* 1986;10: 47–71

41. Davis DL. The meaning of menopause in a Newfoundland fishing village. *Cult Med Psychiatry* 1986;10:73–94

42. George T. Menopause: some interpretations of the results of a study among a non-western group. *Maturitas* 1988;10:109–16

43. Kaiser K. Cross-cultural perspectives on menopause. *Ann N Y Acad Sci* 1990;592:430–2

44. Kay M, Voda A, Olivas G, *et al.* Ethnography of the menopause-related hot flash. *Maturitas* 1982;4:217–27

45. Lock M. Ambiguities of aging: Japanese experience and perceptions of menopause. *Cult Med Psychiatry* 1986;10:23–46

46. Obermeyer CM. Menopause across cultures: a review of the evidence. *Menopause* 2000;7: 184–92

47. Punyahotra S, Dennerstein L, Lehert P. Menopausal experiences of Thai women. Part 1: symptoms and their correlates. *Maturitas* 1997; 26:1–7

48. Hunter MS. Predictors of menopausal symptoms: psychosocial aspects. *Baillieres Clin Endocrinol Metab* 1993;7:33–45

49. Chiazze Jr. L, Brayer FT, Macisco Jr. JJ, *et al.* The length and variability of the human menstrual cycle. *J Am Med Assoc* 1968;203;377–80

50. Bernard JS. *The Female World.* New York: Free Press, 1981

51. Kaufert PA, Gilbert P, Tate R. Defining menopausal status: the impact of longitudinal data. *Maturitas* 1987;9:217–26

52. Depression Guideline Panel. *Depression in Primary Care: Volume 1. Detection and diagnosis* (AHCPR Publication No. 93-0550). Rockville: US Department of Health and Human Services, 1993

53. Depression Guideline Panel. *Depression in Primary Care: Volume 2. Treatment of depression* (AHCPR Publication No. 93-0550). Rockville: US Department of Health and Human Services, 1993

54. Evans MD, Hollon SD, DeRubeis RJ, *et al.* Differential relapse following cognitive therapy and pharmacotherapy for depression. *Arch Gen Psychiatry* 1992;49:802–8

55. Frank E, Grochocinski VJ, Spanier CA, *et al.* Interpersonal psychotherapy and antidepressant medication: evaluation of a sequential treatment strategy in women with recurrent

major depression. *J Clin Psychiatry* 2000;61:51–7

56. Kupfer DJ, Frank E, Perel JM, *et al.* Five-year outcome for maintenance therapies in recurrent depression. *Arch Gen Psychiatry* 1992;49: 769–73

57. Miller IW, Keitner GI. Combined medication and psychotherapy in the treatment of chronic mood disorders. *Psychiatr Clin North Am* 1996; 19:151–71

58. Shea MT, Elkin I, Imber SD, *et al.* Course of depressive symptoms over follow-up: findings from The National Institute of Mental Health Treatment of Depression Collaborative Research program. *Arch Gen Psychiatry* 1992;49:782–7

59. Simon GE, Katon W, Rutter C, *et al.* Impact of improved depression treatment in primary care on daily functioning and disability. *Psychol Med* 1998;28:693–701

60. Magursky V, Mesko M, Sokolik L. Age at the menopause and onset of the climacteric in women of Martin District, Czechoslovakia: statistical survey and some biological and social correlations. *Int J Fertil* 1975;20:17–23

61. McKinlay SM, Brambilla DJ, Posner JG. The normal menopause transition. *Maturitas* 1992; 14:103–15

62. Avis NE, Crawford SL, McKinlay SM. Psychosocial, behavioral and health factors related to menopause symptomatology. *Women's Health: Research on Gender, Behavior and Policy* 1997;3: 103–20

63. McKinlay JB, McKinlay SM, Brambilla D. The relative contributions of endocrine changes and social circumstances to depression in mid-aged women. *J Health Soc Behav* 1987;28:345–63

64. Hunter M, Battersby R, Whitehead M. Relationships between psychological symptoms, somatic complaints and menopausal status. *Maturitas* 1986;8:217–28

65. Kaufert P, Syrotuik J. Symptom reporting at the menopause. *Soc Sci Med* 1981;15E:173–84

66. Dennerstein L, Smith AMA, Morse C, *et al.* Menopausal symptoms in Australian women. *Med J Aust* 1993;159:232–6

67. Dennerstein L, Smith AMA, Morse C. Psychological well-being, mid-life and the menopause. *Maturitas* 1994;20:1–11

68. Winokur G. Depression in the menopause. *Am J Psychiatry* 1973;130:92–3

69. Burt VK, Altshuler LL, Rasgon N. Depressive symptoms in the perimenopause: prevalence, assessment, and guidelines for treatment. *Harv Rev Psychiatry* 1998;6:121–32

70. Schmidt PJ, Nieman L, Danaceau MA, *et al.* Estrogen replacement in perimenopause-related depression: a preliminary report. *Am J Obstet Gynecol* 2000;183:414–20

71. Wilbur J, Dan AJ. The impact of work patterns on psychological well-being of midlife nurses. *West J Nurs Res* 1989;11:703–16

Sexuality

8

M. S. Hunter

INTRODUCTION

In this paper, a general overview of research on sexuality during the climacteric and postmenopause is presented. Definitions of sexual functioning and sexual problems need to be considered within the sociocultural contexts which shape our views and expectations of the sexual functioning of mid-aged and older women. The questions that appear to concern women and men, as well as clinicians, include: what changes across the menopause transition? What factors influence sexual functioning during mid-life? And how are sexual problems, if they do arise, best treated? These questions are addressed in the sections that follow.

DEFINITIONS

Sexuality represents a complex interplay of various physiological, psychosocial and cultural factors. In its broadest sense sexuality embraces a person's gender identity, roles, physical appearance, reproductive potential, sexual feelings and behavior. However, most academic and clinical discussions of sexuality focus upon sexual functioning and sexual dysfunction. Dimensions of sexual functioning typically include:

(1) Sexual desire, interest or libido;

(2) Frequency of sexual activity, such as sexual fantasies and intercourse;

(3) Arousal, reflected by vaginal lubrication, responsiveness, vaginal blood flow;

(4) Orgasm, enjoyment and frequency;

(5) Satisfaction with sexual experiences and with sexual relationship;

(6) Partner's sexual functioning.

Sexual dysfunction is classified by the DSM-IV[1] as a disturbance in the processes that characterize the sexual response cycle (desire, excitement/arousal, orgasm and resolution) or by pain associated with sexual intercourse or dyspareunia (discomfort during penetration). Common problems are reduced libido and reduced arousal, as evidenced in lack of vaginal lubrication and erectile difficulties. Inherent in these definitions is an emphasis on performance, rather than other aspects of sexuality, such as enjoyment. There is also discordance between 'sexual dysfunction' as defined by health professionals and an individual's perceptions of their sexual lives. In other words the relationships between the doctor's and patient's definitions are often quite poor[2]. Sexual problems occur in the context of a relationship and are in practice defined according to the relative perceptions of the couple.

MEASURES OF SEXUAL FUNCTIONING

Several standardized questionnaires have been developed to measures aspects of sexual functioning for men and women, such as the Derogatis Interview Schedule for Sexual Functioning[3] and The Golombok Rust Inventory of Sexual Satisfaction[4]. These measures assess sexual fantasy, arousal, behavior and experience, motivation and aspects of the relationship. The McCoy Female Sexuality Questionnaire[5] is a 19-item scale with five main subscales measuring sexual interest, satisfaction, vaginal lubrication, orgasm and the sexual functioning of the partner. This scale has been widely used in studies of climacteric and postmenopausal women, and shorter versions of the questionnaire exist. Similarly, the Sexual Activities Questionnaire[6] was developed to investigate the long-term impact of tamoxifen in mid-aged women at risk of breast cancer, with a general population comparison group. Using factor analysis the authors grouped items into three main dimensions: sexual pleasure, sexual discomfort and activity. Sexual items are also included in other general scales, for example the Women's Health Questionnaire[7] (developed for mid-aged and older women) and the Cancer Rehabilitation Evaluation System[8] (developed for women who may have menopausal symptoms following cancer treatment). It is advisable to measure specific sexual domains as well as including a more general health related quality of life measure (see Chapters 8 and 9) in epidemiological studies and in assessments of treatment outcomes.

CULTURAL ASSUMPTIONS AND BELIEFS

In the past, and in most cultures, acceptable sexual behavior has been based on the premise that men need and are entitled to sex and that women's sexual pleasure should be secondary to the interests of male enjoyment and reproduction. Consequently, female sexuality has been very much linked to reproduction. The values of the nineteenth century reinforced sexual taboos and inhibitions. There has also tended to be a heterosexual focus in research on sexuality, with an assumption that all women are either heterosexual or want to have a heterosexual relationship.

With the association of female sexuality with youth and reproductive capacity the menopause has been seen as the end of a woman's sexual life[9]. However, these assumptions have been challenged during the past century following changes in attitude to sexuality during the 1960s and the developments of hormonal therapies for climacteric and post-menopausal women. Today, the pendulum has swung in that sexuality is now equated with health and well-being – mid-aged and older women can expect to maintain sexual responsiveness and activity. Thus there are varied – and often conflicting – beliefs about female

Table 1 Methodological problems in epidemiological studies

Selected samples, such as clinics, advertisements
Bias towards educated and sexually active women
Natural versus surgical menopause
Confounding of age and menopausal status
Different measures used
Lack of consideration of the woman's partner

sexuality, particularly relating to older women. It is important that health professionals examine their own assumptions and health beliefs so that they can approach female patients with an open mind and a non-judgmental attitude.

WHAT CHANGES DURING THE MENOPAUSE TRANSITION?

This question is best addressed by well-designed prospective studies using general population samples. Methodological problems abound in this area of research (see Table 1). For example, women attending menopause clinics have been found to report a relatively high prevalence of sexual problems compared to non-clinic samples[9]. Similarly, the type of menopause – surgical or natural – might differentially influence aspects of sexual response. Cross-sectional studies often confound the effects of age as well as cohort effects. Other variables, such as length of relationship, the quality of the relationship and the partner's sexual functioning (if the women has a relationship) need to be taken into account.

A number of cross-sectional studies have been conducted and there is general consensus that, with age, indices of sexual functioning tend to decline for both men and women[10–13]. For example, Kinsey and colleagues[10] interviewed women across the life cycle and found a decline in incidence and frequency of sexual activity (intercourse and orgasm) with age, but not in solitary sexual activity such as masturbation, which continued until well after 60 years. Pfeiffer and co-workers[11] studied women and men aged 46–71 and found a gradual decrease in sexual interest and coital activity with age, particularly between the ages of

45–55, for both men and women. A gradual decrement in measures of sexual functioning during mid-life has been suggested by cross-sectional results, and when the effects of age and menopausal stage have been examined separately there appears to be a small additional effect for menopause over and above age effects on sexual functioning[12,14,15]. For example, in a study carried out in South East England[14] approximately 70% of the 474 women, aged 45–56, reported being sexually active. Sexual interest decreased across the stages of the menopause when the effects of age were controlled, and vaginal dryness was more commonly reported by postmenopausal women. However, 26% of premenopausal women also reported having vaginal dryness; this rose to 46% of postmenopausal women. Despite these changes over 80% of the women reported being satisfied with their current sexual relationship. Similar findings have been reported by other authors[13,15].

McCoy and Davidson[16] carried out the first prospective study of sexual behavior in 16 women. Small but significant decreases in sexual activity, sexual thoughts and vaginal lubrication were found across the menopause transition, but no changes in orgasmic frequency or sexual enjoyment were evident. In a more recent Australian study – the Melbourne Women's Health Project[17] – 354 women aged 45–55 were followed in a six year prospective study. Across time there were declines in reports of libido, responsivity, frequency of sexual activity and feelings for partner. Increases in vaginal dryness and sexual problems in the woman's partner were also reported. Menopausal status had an independent effect on these variables over and above the effects of age.

There is a growing consensus that indices of sexual functioning such as activity and interest decrease across the menopause transition, and that vaginal dryness is more frequently reported by postmenopausal women. However, it is important to view these results in perspective. In most studies there are considerable individual differences between women, and overall approximately 60% of women report no change in sexual functioning[14,15], while 60–80% report no change in their satisfaction with their sexual lives[13,14]. With age, more sexual stimulation is needed for sexual arousal for both sexes. Some couples may adjust to this more effectively than others. In the following sections the relative impact of physiological changes and psychosocial factors will be considered.

PHYSICAL CHANGES AND SEXUALITY

There are marked changes in hormone production during the menopause transition. These include an approximate drop in estrogen production of 85%, a reduction in estrone of 58% and a reduction in testosterone of 29%[18]. Therefore the largest change is in estradiol production and the smallest in testosterone production. In addition, the postmenopausal ovary continues to produce significant amounts of androstenedione and testosterone in approximately 50% of naturally postmenopausal women[19]. On the other hand, ovariectomized women are likely to be androgen deficient.

Changes in sexual functioning during mid-age are commonly attributed to hormonal changes, but recent research suggests that there are specific, rather than global, hormonal effects. There is evidence that lower levels of estrogen are associated with vaginal dryness, reduced vaginal blood flow and dyspareunia, but not other indices of sexual functioning, such as enjoyment, interest or activity. There appears to be a peak of reporting of vaginal dryness and discomfort three years into the postmenopause[20]. However, in a physiological study Laan and van Lunsen[21] challenged the assumption that there is a direct relationship between estrogen and reports of vaginal dryness. They studied 42 naturally postmenopausal women and eight premenopausal women. They compared subjective sexual response, and physiological state (measures of vaginal pulse amplitude, estrogen, androgen and prolactin) while at rest and then in response to erotic fantasy and films. Objective criteria were also used to assess the degree of vaginal atrophy of both groups. Interestingly, the postmenopausal women evidenced lower vaginal blood flow at rest than the premenopausal women, but there was no difference between the groups in response to stimulation. Estrogen was associated with degree of vaginal atrophy but not with reported vaginal dryness or pain. Testosterone levels did not differ between the two groups. Prolactin (a hormone that is elevated under conditions of stress) was the only hormone to be associated with indices of sexual functioning – in particular reduced sexual drive, arousal and lubrication. The authors conclude that complaints of vaginal dryness/dyspareunia may be the result of 'arousal problems' rather than vaginal atrophy *per se*. Furthermore, the association between prolactin and sexual functioning suggests that psychosocial factors may be important in influencing sexual interest and arousal.

Testosterone is generally associated with the motivational aspects of sexuality, for example sexual desire and coital frequency[16]. There is more evidence of the effects of testosterone on sexual interest in women following surgical menopause, than in women who have experienced natural menopause[22]. In a detailed review of the literature on the effects of endogenous and exogenous hormones upon sexuality during the menopause, Myers[23] examined cross-sectional, prospective and treatment studies. He concluded that there were some hormone effects but that overall these were small and that the strongest evidence came from studies of androgens, rather than estrogens, with women who had surgically induced menopause.

Additional physical changes include cessation of menstruation and commonly vasomotor symptoms, such as hot flushes and night sweats. For women who have experienced premenstrual symptoms, or menorrhagia (heavy menstruation), or who have found contraception problematic, becoming post-menopausal might be welcomed as a positive influence upon sexual functioning. Approximately 60–70% of women experience vasomotor symptoms, while 15–20% of women report that they are difficult to deal with[24]. Having frequent and intense night sweats can interfere with general physical comfort and

Table 2 Factors influencing sexual functioning during mid-life

Age
Quality of relationship with partner
Physical and emotional health
Partner's sexual functioning
Psychosocial stress
Menopausal symptoms
Past sexual behavior
Length of relationship
Beliefs and expectations
Partner availability

sexual desire and thus impair sexual functioning[17]. Furthermore, ill health causing pain and disability, and medications – for example some antidepressants – can have a negative impact upon sexual functioning. Fear of pain or exacerbation of health problems is not uncommon following diagnoses and treatment for cancer and cardiovascular disease. Ill-health can also lead to a change in roles between couples, for example one partner becoming more dependent upon the other, which could have a negative effect on the relationship. Among women aged over 65 years, one of the major reasons for reduced sexual interest and activity is ill health[25].

PSYCHOSOCIAL INFLUENCES ON SEXUALITY

There is now considerable evidence from epidemiological studies that psychosocial factors, such as variables associated with age, relationship with partner, partner availability, past sexual functioning, mood, stress, beliefs and social situation, account for most of the variation in measures of sexual functioning[13,15–17] (see Table 2). For example, in Hawton's community study in the UK of 436 women aged 35–59[13], age (of the woman and her partner), length of the relationship and the quality of the marital relationship were the main predictors of the frequency of sexual activity. Indeed, aging and length of relationship are known to affect the sexual functioning of both men and women. For example, in a cross-sectional and prospective study, James[26] found that during the first year of marriage the frequency of sexual intercourse halved, and then halved again over the subsequent 20 years. It is important not to evaluate sexual functioning according to frequency alone, since, despite these changes, the majority (60–70%) of the women in Hawton's study reported being satisfied with their current sexual relationship. Similarly, in another cross-sectional UK study, sexual functioning was most strongly associated with marital satisfaction, stress, ill-health and menopausal status. In the prospective phase of this study the main predictors of sexual interest and enjoyment during the menopause were sexual functioning and reported stress *before* the menopause[27]. However, again the majority evaluated their sexual relationships as being satisfactory.

Emotional problems and stressful life events can have adverse effects on sexual feelings. For example, anxiety inhibits sexual arousal and loss of libido is a commonly reported symptom of depression. Similarly, being overly tired as a result of physical or emotional problems can have a negative influence upon sexual relationships. Low self-esteem, particularly if a women takes on board negative social stereotypes about being menopausal, can make her feel less interesting and less sexually attractive. Sociodemographic factors such as employment status and educational level have been associated with sexual functioning, as has having a psychiatric history, and may reflect preoccupation with psychosocial problems[12,13].

The quality of a premenopausal woman's sexual relationship does seem to be one of the main predictors of sexual functioning during and after the menopause. There is also some evidence to suggest that regular and continued sexual activity appears to protect against the development of vaginal dryness[28]. Similarly, it is not surprising that marital satisfaction, or the quality of the relationship which includes communication, ability to show affection and adjust to life changes as well as sexual changes with age, is a strong predictor of sexual functioning. Partner variables had for many years been neglected in studies of women's sexuality. It is now recognized that the male partner's health and sexual functioning play an equal role. In addition, partner availability is a particular issue for older women; the availability of partners decreases for women as they age. In the USA it is estimated that among the over 65s there are approximately four single women for every one male. In this age group the major reasons for decline in sexual interest and activity are ill-health and lack of available partner[25].

Cultural beliefs and values are important influences upon expectations of sexual functioning in mid-age and later life. For example, religious beliefs that sexual activity serves only a procreational purpose may make discussion of sexuality difficult after the menopause. Some couples may regard the sexual aspects of their relationship as less significant as they age and therefore be quite happy with reduced sexual contact. For others, for example those who have begun new relationships, sexual activity may be more highly valued. Good communication and sensitivity are likely to be important in a couple's adjustment to the changes that can affect sexual functioning occurring with age for both sexes. Indeed, it is often the case that problems arise when there is a desynchrony in the needs and expectations between the individuals in a couple.

The relative contributions of hormonal and psychosocial influences upon sexual functioning in women during the menopause transition were examined in detail in the Melbourne Women's Health Project[17]. Structural equation modeling (a type of regression analysis) was used to explore the interrelationships between variables such as age, hormonal status (estrogen, follicle stimulating hormone, inhibin), menopausal status, psychosocial factors and relationship factors, and indices of sexual functioning, measured by the Personal Experiences Questionnaire (a modified version of the McCoy Female Sexuality Questionnaire[5], assessing sexual responsivity, vaginal dryness/dyspareunia, libido and sexual activity). Three hundred and fifty-four women, aged 45–55 years, were followed in a six year prospective study. There was a 90% retention rate across time points. The main factors affecting sexuality were:

(1) Feelings for partner and partner's sexual functioning – these variables had direct effects upon sexual responsivity and libido, and indirect effects upon sexual functioning by influencing women's well-being;

(2) Well-being was influenced by stress, education and employment and had direct effects upon sexual responsivity, which in turn influenced the frequency of sexual activity and libido;

(3) The experience of vasomotor symptoms was influenced, as expected, by menopausal status and again had direct effects upon sexual responsivity, and hence sexual activity and libido;

(4) Menopausal status had direct effects upon vaginal dryness and dyspareunia, and indirect effects upon sexual responsivity, via vasomotor symptoms;

(5) Hormones had no direct effects on sexual functioning. However, there were indirect effects upon measures of sexual functioning which were mediated by the impact of hormones upon menopausal status. In this way hormones had indirect effects upon vaginal dryness and dyspareunia and responsivity.

The authors concluded that the effects of hormones are relatively weak. Moreover, there was no significant relationship in this study between hormone replacement therapy use and sexual functioning. The main factors impacting upon sexual functioning during the menopause transition were feelings for partner, partner problems, well-being and experience of menopausal symptoms. Vaginal dryness and dyspareunia were directly influenced by menopausal status, but there may be additional arousal problems as suggested earlier[21]. The results of this study suggest that it is helpful to breakdown the dimensions of sexual functioning and the range of possible influences. These are likely to differ between individual women and couples and therefore treatment, if warranted, could be tailored to these specific needs.

TREATMENTS FOR SEXUAL PROBLEMS DURING MIDLIFE

When a mid-aged woman seeks help for a sexual problem a detailed history should be taken focusing upon the woman alone, her partner and the couple together. The problem needs to be understood within the context of the relationship, the needs and expectations of both individuals and the range of factors influencing sexual functioning outlined above. Given the relative importance of partner factors over that of hormonal factors, it makes sense to explore these and to adopt a biopsychosocial model in the assessment of sexual difficulties, which gives equal emphasis to psychological, social and biological factors. Specific treatments have a role, for example hormone treatment for vasomotor symptoms, but commonly problems result from relationship difficulties and other stresses in people's lives. The main treatments for psychosexual problems experienced during the menopause transition include hormonal treatments and couple therapy.

Hormone replacement therapy does help vaginal dryness and pain but has no significant effect upon other indices of sexual functioning. Indirect improvements may result from the alleviation of hot flushes and night sweats, if these have been disruptive. There is evidence supporting the use of androgens for women who have experienced surgical menopause; Sherwin and colleagues reported higher rates of sexual desire, sexual arousal and number of sexual fantasies in women who received combined estrogen–androgen therapy than in women who were either given estrogen only or who were untreated[22,29]. Similarly, there is some evidence that tibolone, which is metabolized to three major metabolites with different estrogenic, progestogenic and androgenic properties, may have beneficial effects on sexual functioning – such as reduced vaginal dryness and increased libido – but further research is needed[30,31].

Couple therapy can include assessment with brief intervention focusing upon communication and information and adopting a psychoeducational approach. For example, this might improve communication and adaptation to normal physiological changes. It can also involve assessment and several treatment sessions to explore and help couples to deal with particular identified problems, such as communication, problem-solving life stresses, expressing needs and particular sexual difficulties[32].

An important role for the health professional is to help couples make sense of their problems within a biopsychosocial framework, emphasizing changes in sexual functioning with age for both sexes and the important effects of life stresses, ill-health and communication for the couple. With helpful information presented in a constructive manner, men and women can be helped to adjust to such changes and, given the opportunity, improvements to sexual enjoyment can be made.

A common interpretation of a sexual problem is that there is something very wrong with the relationship. This can lead to feelings of rejection and withdrawal. If it is more appropriate to attribute reduced sexual desire, for example, to tiredness or work stress, then this can enable possible solutions to be found that do not feed into a negative cycle. There may be different expectations and preferences for, say, the frequency of sexual activity between two people in a couple. This needs to be acknowledged without making either person feel that they are the cause of a problem. Once reframed as a difference in preference then the issue can be negotiated. Many couples are reassured when given the opportunity to verbalize their feelings towards one another. For example, if sexual activity has been difficult due to ill-health, in a relationship in which intimacy and affection was focused on sexual activity, the individuals might feel distanced and rejected when this channel of communication is withdrawn. Discussion of this sequence of events can enable couples to communicate their feelings verbally, which is usually reassuring. A psychoeducational approach can include a discussion of the many and varied influences upon sexuality during midlife, as described above and examined in the Melbourne

Women's Health Project. An examination of the relative contribution of these factors for both partners and for the couple can then inform the choice of intervention. In most cases clarification and problem solving is adequate. For example, if night sweats are identified as the main problem, help can be given to alleviate these. If ill health or life stress, such as bereavement, has led to depression and tiredness, then intervention can focus upon increasing relaxation and pleasant activities, and negotiating the kind of sexual contact that the couple feel is helpful in the circumstances.

Some women, having found relief from the cessation of menstruation and contraception after the menopause may feel they want to enjoy a more fulfilling sexual relationship. Making changes in long-term relationships can be difficult, so having the opportunity to talk about their needs and desires in a non-judgmental atmosphere can facilitate positive changes. Some people hold beliefs that can lead to further problems, such as "If we love each other then sex should always be fine." This belief is likely to lead to a more devastating emotional reaction to any sexual difficulty, than a belief such as "Many factors can affect sexual feelings and these are likely to vary across the life-span." Couples' beliefs and expectations about their sexual lives after the menopause can be discussed; negative social stereotypes can be challenges, such as "You have to be young and beautiful to be sexually attractive."

Specific problems such as depression or anxiety can be referred to a specialist for medication and/or psychological treatment, such as cognitive behavior therapy. Psychosexual counseling[32] is helpful for a range of problems, such as reduced sexual desire and erectile impotence. Initially, this approach concentrates upon communication and clarification of needs and then moves on to gradual exploration of what is pleasurable for one another. There may be barriers that are identified during the process of treatment, such as particular fears, which can then be identified and explored. Most couples who seek help are motivated to improve their relationships. However, if there are considerable problems in a relationship then it could be predictable that there would be sexual problems. The options of marital counseling or individual psychological support can be discussed.

For some women the menopause occurs unexpectedly and can be more difficult to adjust to. Early menopause can confront women at a young age with problems such as vaginal dryness which are difficult to understand and accept. It is also common for these women to believe that they are suddenly aging. As well as having to deal with physical changes they are also faced with negative social stereotypes about the menopause at a young age. As a result self-esteem can be adversely affected. Treating menopausal symptoms and helping these women to adjust, while at the same time challenging unhelpful beliefs, can help them to maintain some continuity on their sense of identity[33].

Premature menopause is also a common consequence of many cancer treatments. Chemotherapy and/or radiation may damage the gonadal–pituitary axis and result in early menopause. Similarly, tamoxifen treatment for the prevention of breast cancer produces menopausal symptoms, hot flushes and night sweats in at least 57% of those taking it[34]. Psychosexual functioning was examined in a study comparing survivors of breast cancer, who had undergone a range of treatments and who had been prescribed hormone replacement therapy. These women were compared with age- and socioeconomic-status-matched controls, using the Derogatis Sexual Functioning Inventory[35]. Eighty-two per cent of the sample reported concerns about their sexual functioning and a significantly greater proportion of this group (39%) reported sexual difficulties, particularly low sexual desire. The presence of menopausal symptoms and relationship adjustment were the main predictors of sexual problems in this sample, despite their hormonal treatment. The authors suggest that further clinical interventions need to be developed for these women. In a recent study, Ganz and colleagues[36] evaluated the effectiveness of a comprehensive menopausal

assessment (CMA) intervention program with the aims of relieving symptoms and improving quality of life and sexual functioning in breast cancer survivors. The intervention was delivered by a nurse practitioner and focused upon symptom assessment, education, counseling and, as appropriate, specific pharmacological and behavioral interventions such as vaginal lubricants, relaxation exercises and individual and group counseling. Sexual functioning was assessed using the Sexual Functioning Scale of the Cancer Rehabilitation Evaluation System, and the SF-36 (Vitality Scale) was used to measure quality of life. After four months of treatment the intervention group demonstrated significant improvements in menopausal symptoms and sexual functioning, but no difference on the Vitality (SF-36) assessing quality of life, compared to a control group receiving usual care.

This study raises the question of the relationship between reports of sexual difficulties and health related quality of life in general. The point was made earlier that having low sexual desire, for example, does not in itself mean that the person or couple have a sexual problem – rather the appraisal of a person's sexual functioning is very personal and can only be defined as problematic by them in the context of their relationship. In the same way sexual functioning may impact on quality of life but not necessarily. It is therefore as important when assessing sexual functioning to ask about the person's individual appraisal of the 'problem' and whether it is seen to be a problem for them.

CONCLUSIONS

A broader perspective on sexuality is needed that includes sexual functioning but also enjoyment and a general appraisal of a sexual relationship. While in epidemiological studies a decrement in many areas of sexual functioning is apparent, considerable individual differences exist, such that it is very difficult to generalize from such studies to the individual case. Menopause is not, contrary to popular belief, universally associated with diminished sexual activity: some women report a decrease, others an increase. For the majority (60%) there is little change in sexual functioning, and it is important to remember that the majority report being satisfied with their sexual relationships despite changes in sexual functioning.

Similarly, it is important for health professionals to be aware of their own assumptions and beliefs about the sexuality of mid-aged and older women, and men. Particularly it is helpful not to assume heterosexuality, or that sexual activity is necessarily associated with quality of life. Instead it makes sense to sensitively explore if there is a problem and with whom, and to let the couple define whether a change in sexual functioning is problematic. Moreover, some people may wish to discuss a problem that is concerning them but be too embarrassed to do so. Therefore it helps to discuss sexuality in the context of the menopause and to acknowledge that some women experience changes, positive and negative, while others do not. There is a need to focus on both men and women when considering sexual functioning of mid-aged and older couples. Contrary to previously held beliefs, sexual problems occurring during the menopause transition do not always rest with the woman.

While hormonal changes can have specific – although relatively weak – effects on sexual functioning, largely mediated by their influence on vasomotor symptoms and vaginal dryness, aging and psychosocial influences account for most of the variation in sexual functioning during this life stage (see Table 2). Detailed assessment is needed examining a wide range of influences for both partners in a couple. Following this a specific intervention can be planned, if this is wanted, which is tailored to these particular needs. Again it is important not to assume that everyone acknowledging a problem in response to questions wishes to have treatment. Some people want information and advice and in the context of the menopause and age changes, brief interventions (which might include information, facilitating communication about needs, advice about dealing with symptoms and stress) can be very helpful. There is also a role for health education[37] and preparation for events, such as surgery and medical treatments, which may impact upon sexual functioning.

References

1. *Diagnostic and Statistical Manual of Mental Disorders*, Fourth Edition. Washington: American Psychiatric Association, 493–4

2. Osborne M, Hawton K, Gath D. Sexual dysfunction among middle-aged women in the community. *BMJ* 1988;296:959–62

3. Derogatis LR, Melisaratos N. The DSFI: a multidimensional measure of sexual functioning. *J Sex Marital Ther* 1997;5:244–81

4. Golombok S, Rust J. The Golombok Rust Inventory of Sexual Satisfaction. Berkshire: NFER-Nelson, 1986

5. McCoy N. The McCoy Female Sexuality Questionnaire. *Qual Life Res* 2001;9:739–45

6. Thirlaway K, Fallowfield L, Cuzick J. The Sexual Activity Questionnaire: a measure of women's sexual functioning. *Qual Life Res* 1996;5:81–90

7. Hunter MS. The Women's Health Questionnaire: a measure of mid-aged women's perceptions of their emotional and physical health. *Psychol Health* 1992;7:45–54

8. Ganz PA, Schag CA, Lee JJ, *et al.* The CARES: a generic measure of health related quality of life for patients with cancer. *Qual Life Res* 1992;1:19–29

9. Sarrel P, Whitehead MI. Sex and menopause: defining the issues. *Maturitas* 1985;7:217–24

10. Kinsey AC, Pomeroy WB, Martin CE, *et al.* Sexual behaviour in the human female. Saunders: Philadelphia, 1983:734–6

11. Pfeiffer E, Vervoerdt A, Davis GC. Sexual behaviour in middle life. *Am J Psychiatry* 1972;128:1262–7

12. Hallstrom T. Sexuality of women in middle age: the Goteborg study. *J Biosoc Sci* 1979;6:165–75

13. Hawton K, Gath D, Day A. Sexual function in a community sample of middle-aged women with partners: effects of age, marital, socioeconomic, psychiatric, gynaecological and menopausal factor. *Arch Sex Behav* 1994;23:375–95

14. Hunter MS. Emotional well-being, sexual behaviour and hormone replacement therapy. *Maturitas* 1990;12:299–314

15. Dennerstein L, Smith AMA, Morse CA, *et al.*

Sexuality and the menopause. *J Psychosom Obstet Gynecol* 1994;15:59–66

16. McCoy N, Davidson JM. A longitudinal study of the effects of menopause on sexuality. *Maturitas* 1985;7:203–10

17. Dennerstein L, Lehert P, Burger H, *et al.* Factors affecting sexual functioning of women in the middle years. *Climacteric* 1999;2,254–62

18. Longcope C, Jaffe W, Griffing G. Production rates of androgens and oestrogens in postmenopausal women. *Maturitas* 1981;3:215–23

19. Longcope C, Hunter R, Franz C. Steroid secretion by the postmenopausal ovary. *Am J Obstet Gynecol* 1980;138:564–8

20. Holte A. Influences of natural menopause on health complaints: a prospective study of healthy Norwegian women. *Maturitas* 1992;14:127–41

21. Laan E, van Lunsen RHW. Hormones and sexuality in postmenopausal women: a psychophysiological study. *J Psychosom Obstet Gynecol* 1997;18:126–33

22. Sherwin BB, Gelfand MM, Brender W. Androgen enhances motivation in females: a prospective, crossover study of sex steroid administration in the surgical menopause. *Psychosom Med* 1985;47:339–51

23. Myers L. Methodological review and meta-analysis of sexuality and menopause research. *Neurosci Biobehav Rev* 1995;19:331–41

24. Hunter MS, Liao KLM. A psychological analysis of menopausal hot flushes. *Br J Clin Psychol* 1995;34:589–99

25. Roughan PA, Kaiser FE, Morley JE. Sexuality and the older woman. *Clinics Geriatric Med* 1993; 9:87–106

26. James W. Decline in coital rates with spouse's ages in duration of marriage. *J Biosoc Sci* 183;15: 83–7

27. Hunter MS. Predictors of menopausal symptoms; psychological aspects. In Burger HG, ed. *The Menopause. Bailliere's Clinical Endocrinology and Metabolism.* London: Bailliere Tindall, 1993: 33–46

28. Leiblum SR, Bachmann GA, Kemman E, *et al.* Vaginal atrophy in the postmenopausal woman. *J Am Med Assoc* 1983;249:2195–8

29. Sherwin BB. Use of combined estrogen preparations in the postmenopause: evidence from clinical studies. *Int J Fertil* 1998;29:41–50

30. Moore RA. Livial: a review of clinical studies. *Br J Obstet Gynaecol* 1999;106:1–21

31. Rymer J, Chapman MG, Fogelman I, *et al.* A study of the effect of tibolone on the vagina in postmenopausal women. *Maturitas* 1994;18: 127–33

32. Bancroft J. *Human Sexuality and its Problems.* Edinburgh: Churchill Livingstone, 1989

33. Singer D, Hunter M, eds. *Premature Menopause: A Multidisciplinary Approach.* London: Whurr, 2000:232–50

34. Fisher B, Costantino J, Redmond C, *et al.* A randomized clinical trial evaluating tamoxifen in the treatment of patients with node-negative breast cancer who have estrogen receptor positive tumours. *N Engl J Med* 1989;320:479–84

35. Moadel AB, Ostroff JS, Lesko LM, *et al.* Psychosexual adjustment among women receiving hormone replacement therapy for premature menopause following cancer treatment. *Psychooncology* 1995;4:273–82

36. Ganz PA, Greendale GA, Peterson L, *et al.* Managing symptoms in breast cancer survivors: results of a randomised controlled trial. *J Natl Cancer Inst* 2000;92:1054–64

37. Hunter MS, O'Dea I. An evaluation of a health education intervention for mid-aged women: five year follow-up of effects upon knowledge, impact of menopause and health. *Patient Educ Counsel* 1999;38:249–55

The cost-effectiveness and cost-utility of hormone replacement therapy 9

Y. F. Zöllner

LEARNING OBJECTIVES

The aim of this chapter is two-fold. Firstly, it shall familiarize the reader with the terms, concepts and methods used in health economics, thus providing the necessary background knowledge to understand and interpret original health economic research papers. The chronological approach is intended to reflect the development of both health economics as a discipline and hormone treatment strategies of postmenopausal women. Secondly, the chapter shall review the key health economic studies in the field of menopause and hormone replacement therapy (HRT) published to date, highlighting their relative strengths and weaknesses.

HEALTH ECONOMICS

Why is health economics relevant?

Faced with the increasing cost of healthcare provision, many governments have sought new policy options to contain expenditure. One of the drivers of healthcare expenditure has been the rapid rate of technological advance in pharmaceuticals in recent years and the prices charged for new medicines.

A number of rationing devices have been introduced – with varying degrees of success – to contain pharmaceutical expenditure, including patient co-payments, physician prescription budgets (in some cases with incentives to under-spend and sanctions for over-spending), reference prices, de-reimbursement, prescription guidelines and formularies. Figure 1 reflects the development of public pharmaceutical expenditure from 1980 to 1996 in various OECD countries.

Many pharmaceuticals have been subject to economic evaluation in the past, but this has largely been unsystematic and with no firm policy objective. In recent years, however, policy-makers have been looking at economic evaluation as a basis to inform resource allocation decisions. It has been suggested that there is considerable scope for extending the current use of economics in pricing and reimbursement decisions. A growing number of countries have encouraged economic evaluation of new medicines to ensure that only medicines proven to be both clinically effective and economically viable are reimbursed or made available on formularies. Some countries, in an attempt to overcome the problems surrounding interpretability and applicability of the evidence, have introduced formal pharmaco-economic guidelines – a set of rules for the economic evaluation of pharmaceuticals[1].

Cost-effectiveness has not been used as a criterion for marketing approval to date, but rather has influenced the decision to reimburse new medicines. This approach is often referred to as the 'fourth hurdle', implying cost-effectiveness is an additional hurdle to market, complementing safety, efficacy and pharmaceutical quality. Table 1 reflects the role of economic evaluation of pharmaceuticals for different policy objectives in various countries.

What can health economics do?

Health economics can be defined as the application of the theories, tools and concepts

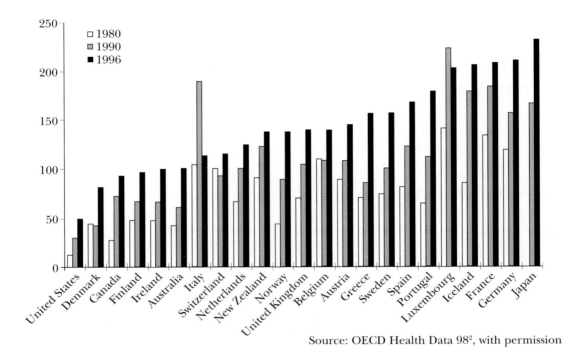

Source: OECD Health Data 98[2], with permission

Figure 1 Public expenditure on pharmaceutical goods per capita. Constant US dollars, current exhange rates

Table 1 Use of pharmaco-economic evaluations for different purposes in selected countries, adapted with permission from Graf von der Schulenburg and Hoffmann, 2000[4]

	Reimbursement	Pricing	Local formulary listing	Development of clinical practice guidelines	Communication to prescribers
Australia	+	+	+	+	+
Belgium	+		+		
Canada	+		+	+	+
Denmark			+	+	+
Finland	+	+		+	
France	+	+			
Germany			+	+	+
Italy	+				
Netherlands	+		+	+	+
Norway	+	+			+
Portugal	+				+
Spain	+				
Sweden	+	+		+	+
Switzerland	+	+			
United Kingdom			+	+	+
United States			+	+	+

of economics to the topics of healthcare. Just as economics is the science of allocating scarce resources to unlimited wants, health economics is concerned with the allocation of scarce health service resources to unlimited demands or needs.

Health technology assessment (HTA), or health economic evaluation, is a sub-discipline of health economics and provides the necessary tools to decide whether a given medical technology is worth funding or not. Economic evaluation aims to identify, measure, value and compare the costs and the outcomes of alternative courses of medical action. Economic evaluation is therefore concerned with both the costs and consequences of treatment alternatives. It is not about choosing the cheapest price alternative, but is designed to identify the alternative that gives greatest value for money. However, economics – and by extension, health economics – is a 'positive' rather than a 'normative' science: it is descriptive rather than prescriptive in nature. Decision-makers may have other than solely economic criteria to inform their decisions, including political, ethical and logistic concerns.

Regarding the economic decision criterion, HTA-driven answers to resource allocation problems can be based on two distinct approaches. The first is an 'implicit approach'. Here, healthcare interventions that compete for scarce resources are ranked in terms of their cost-effectiveness ratio (CER) – the ratio of net costs divided by net effects. The lower the CER, the more favorable the corresponding intervention. Alternative treatment strategies are ranked from best to worst (i.e. lowest to highest) CER, constituting a so-called league table. The decision of whether or not to reimburse a given technology is implicit in its relative position with regard to a critical (i.e. threshold or cut-off) CER. The cut-off CER is typically fixed by the last intervention in the table still considered worth funding. The decision rule is then to promote those programs above and to discourage those below the threshold intervention. However, the determination of the latter is essentially arbitrary and largely based on human

judgment, as the question "what is a reasonable price to pay for a unit of effect?" has no absolute answer. Decisions based on CERs can hence only achieve 'technical efficiency' (as opposed to 'allocative efficiency'). This assumes choosing the intervention that will minimize the cost for a given unit of outcome (or maximize outcome subject to a given budget), without being certain whether the intervention itself is worth funding at all. As an example, genetic testing, which provides information not about actual cancer, but risk of future (breast) cancer, could be technically efficient in that sense. However, its systematic use in screening might not be an altogether wise allocation of resources[3].

The second is an 'explicit approach', embedded in the technique of cost-benefit analysis (CBA). Rather than focusing on ratios and comparing them to each other, CBA provides an absolute answer to the question of whether a treatment is worth funding. Only those interventions whose benefits outweigh their associated costs are eligible for reimbursement. In other words, the health economic requirement for treatments is to produce an overall net benefit, which is operationalized as 'net present value' (NPV), or discounted net benefits minus discounted net costs (discounting is explained in the final paragraph). The decision rule 'implement if NPV > 0' can achieve allocative efficiency, which is superior to the mere technical efficiency mentioned above.

Allocative efficiency, as the name implies, ensures optimal overall allocation of health-care resources. However, CBA requires health outcomes to be valued in monetary terms, an issue over which current controversies are not resolved. Typically, money values are placed on health outcomes either by a patient's willingness to pay (WTP) for a given benefit[5], or by his or her production loss in the absence of health gain. The obvious challenges inherent in these valuation methods have sparked controversies that are still unresolved to date. Medical audiences especially are hesitant to accept this form of analysis. Therefore, the CBAs of HRT, despite some

Table 2 Comparison of cost-effectiveness and cost-utility analysis

	Therapy outcome	*Unit*	*Type of analysis*
Without QoL adjustment	Life expectancy (LE)	Life years (LYs) saved	Cost-effectiveness analysis (CEA)
With QoL adjustment	Quality-adjusted life expectancy (QALE)	Quality-adjusted life years (QALYs) gained	Cost-utility analysis (CUA)

existing studies, are not further discussed in this chapter.

Turning back to the implicit approach and technical efficiency, we summarize that the CER of a healthcare intervention measures its ability to produce improved health outcomes at a reasonable price, which implies comparison to other healthcare interventions. The underlying type of analysis can take one of two forms: (1) cost-effectiveness analysis (CEA), where outcomes are measured in clinical units (such as avoided fractures or infarctions, or years of life saved); or (2) cost-utility analysis (CUA) where potentially all relevant outcomes of therapy are summarized in one single unit or index, usually the quality-adjusted life year (QALY). The latter is a very useful construct that combines the remaining life expectancy with the quality of life (QoL) experienced during those years. That is, when estimating QALYs, not every year of life is weighted equally; instead, each year is assigned a 'preference weight' (QoL weight, utility score) that reflects its value on a scale where 0 represents death and 1 represents perfect health. Typically, the artificial unit 'utils' is used in this context. To illustrate this, ten life-years (LYs) lived at a QoL score of 0.9 utils would correspond to $10 \times 0.9 = 9$ QALYs.

Some authors consider CUA a particular subtype of CEA where life expectancy (LE, in life years) as a non-weighted outcome is quality-adjusted to yield quality-adjusted life expectancy (QALE) expressed in QALY units. However, CUA should really be treated separately, especially in economic appraisals of HRT. CUA is extraordinarily suitable for interventions such as HRT for two reasons: firstly, for the multiplicity of effects of HRT, which make a single outcome index very desirable and secondly for its preventive nature. Preventive treatments characteristically generate costs in the present and near future, but yield benefits only in the distant future. In order to account for the differential timing of costs and benefits, economists often use the technique of discounting. This allows future costs and effects to be translated into 'present values'. Future QALYs are quite amenable to discounting, with one QALY to be gained in 10 years' time translating to a present value of only $1/(1+0.05)^{10} = 0.6$ QALY, using a standard 5% discount rate.

Finally, CUA has the great advantage of allowing comparisons across treatments and is increasingly encouraged by regulatory authorities around the world[4]. A comparison of CEA and CUA is shown in Table 2.

HEALTH ECONOMICS OF HRT

This section will integrate the best available health economic evidence to address the cost-effectiveness and cost-utility of HRT. Given the scope of the book, most attention will be paid to CUA. However, CEA and CUA tend to go hand-in-hand as authors would often relate costs, for the sake of comparison, to both unadjusted and quality-adjusted life-years saved within the same study. The impact and importance of QoL adjustments is thus illustrated. CEAs that relate costs to single outcomes – such as averted fractures – are deemed of too narrow a focus in this context and can be found elsewhere[6].

Early models: data paucity, tentative assumptions

The seminal study, published in 1980, was by

| **Benefits** | fracture prevention (hip and wrist) |
| | symptom relief (where applicable) |

Risks	endometrial carcinoma
	gallbladder disease
	uterine bleeding

Costs	*direct costs*
	Treatment (conjugated estrogens 0.625 mg; two physician visits per year)
	Biopsy (optional)
	induced costs
	Hysterectomy, radiotherapy (endometrial carcinoma)
	Dilatation and curretage (uterine bleeding)
	Cholecystectomy (gallbladder disease)
	induced savings
	Hip fracture prevention
	Wrist fracture prevention

QoL adjustments	symptoms:	minus 0.01 QALY per year of symptom suffering (1%)
	spinal compression fracture:	minus 0.01 QALY for each year of remaining LE (1%)
	hip fracture:	minus 0.05 QALY for each year of remaining LE (5%)
	endometrial cancer:	minus 1 QALY off remaining LE if experienced (0.2 per year, for an average of five years, due to trauma and anxiety)

Box 1 Endpoints included in the original CE model. Remaining life expectancy (LE) is quality-adjusted by subtracting the corresponding QALY estimate of the event where it occurs. Symptomatic women on ERT will increase their quality-adjusted life expectancy (QALE) increased by 0.01 QALY (about four days) per year of treatment.

Milton Weinstein[7]. He was a pioneer in the field of health economics and evidence-based medicine. Given the state of the discipline at the time, the results of the analysis need to be interpreted with care in the current context. However, it is still mentioned here for didactic purposes. The treatment considered is un-opposed estrogen replacement therapy (ERT), quite common-place at that time even for women with intact uteri. Hysterectomy rate was estimated at 30%. The underlying decision–analytic model builds on LE estimates taken from US 1959–61 life tables, and reports various cost-per-QALY ratios for the comparison of ERT with no treatment. The covered endpoints are summarized in Box 1.

Cardiovascular protection is ignored in the model, as is the potential risk of breast cancer. Gallbladder disease, which appeared to be causally associated to estrogen replacement, is accounted for with a relative risk (RR) of 2.5 over non-users of ERT. Fracture data was quite scarce at the time and had to be taken from epidemiologic surveys. QoL adjustments were an absolute novelty and no empirical data were available at the time. Hence, the author himself was the source of utility values assigned to postmenopausal health states.

The author suggests a number of tentative conclusions. Firstly, in hysterectomized women – either symptomatic, osteoporotic or both – ERT would be highly cost-effective due to the absence of risk of endometrial cancer or uterine bleeding, and the lack of need for endometrial biopsies. Secondly, in symptomatic women with intact uteri, ERT was found to be cost-effective for those women at high risk of osteoporosis; for those at average risk of osteoporosis, the cost-effectiveness of treatment was found to hinge heavily on the subjective importance attached to the attenuation of symptoms. ERT did not appear

Table 3 Cost per quality-adjusted life-years gained with ERT as opposed to no therapy (1979 US dollars)

	Non-hysterectomized women	Hysterectomized women
Symptomatic women	$7400*	$4800
Women with clinical osteoporosis	$5500*	$3250

Treatment duration is assumed to be ten years (age 50–60) for symptomatic women and 15 years (age 55–70) for osteoporotic women; *assumes no annual biopsy

Table 4 Cost per quality-adjusted life-years gained with combined HRT under central assumptions

	Combined estrogen–progestogen therapy, treatment duration		
	50–55 years	50–60 years	50–65 years
Compared to 'no treatment'	$42 000 ($20 000)	$29 000 ($17 000)	$24 000 ($15 000)
Compared to 'estrogen-only'	$33 400*	$6500*	$5600*

CERs if periodic bleeding was assumed to confer no loss in QoL are shown in brackets (1982 US dollars); *assuming no biopsies on ERT

to be cost-effective as a prophylactic measure in asymptomatic women, with or without a uterus. Adding up incurred costs and savings to address the net budget impact of wide ERT prescription, he concludes that these would come close to cancelling each other out (cost-neutrality). However, he highlights that "the cost-effectiveness of estrogen use at the societal level depends critically on the subjective values assigned to symptomatic relief".

This under-researched area was to be neglected for a further decade, but it gradually became incorporated into subsequent health economic assessments of HRT.

Three years later, Weinstein and Schiff[8] amended and re-ran their model comparing combined estrogen–progestogen with estrogen-only and no therapy. The model built on the structure proposed in 1980 now featured three additional endpoints: endometrial hyperplasia, breast cancer and cardiovascular disease. Moreover, the incidence and risk data for hip and wrist fracture were taken from newer studies. A further (but optional) QoL assumption to those previously outlined is that any symptomatic benefit will be reduced by one-half when a progestogen is added, in order to account for the effect of continued menstruation. Regarding its net economic impact, they found that with the progestogen (here: medroxyprogesterone acetate, MPA) added, the reduced costs of endometrial monitoring and treatment of endometrial lesions more than offset the increased cost of the drug regimen – with a net saving of $US 230–430 per patient, depending on the duration of treatment (cost-saving). Further-more, the combined therapy is estimated to increase life expectancy by one month, relative to no treatment, if continued on a long-term basis, owing to the reduction in hip fractures, and despite the possible risk of breast cancer.

The authors concluded that combination therapy is highly cost-effective, particularly if endometrial biopsies were omitted, if therapy continued for ≥ 10 years, and if QoL was unchanged by periodic bleeding. Under these conditions, cost per QALY could be as little as $US 5600 (in 1982 US dollars) for 15 years of treatment (Table 3).

To illustrate the cost-effectiveness of combined HRT relative to other interventions, the authors pointed out that under the central assumptions, the CER of combined HRT

Table 5 Cost per quality-adjusted life year gained with various hormone replacement strategies (1988 US dollars) according to the Weinstein and Tosteson model[9] (reproduced with permission from the *Annals of the New York Academy of Sciences*)

	Effect of treatment on quality of life				
	–0.5%	*0%*	*+0.5%*	*+1%*	*+2%*
E alone, 5 years	*	72 100	33 100	21 500	12 600
E+P, 5 years	59 700	26 100	16 700	12 300	8000
E+P, 15 years	30 600	24 000	19 700	16 700	12 800

E, estrogen; P, progestogen; *net effectiveness is negative (loss of QALE), hence negative CER.

compared favourably to the CER for treatment of moderate diastolic hypertension. At the same time, the authors emphasize that the comparison between the two treatments in terms of QALE – or QALYs generated throughout the remaining LE – critically depended on the magnitude of the perceived reduction in QoL caused by progestogen-induced periodic bleeding.

In a follow-up study, Weinstein and Tosteson[9] refined the 1983 model, re-populating it with newly emerged data on the epidemiology of bone mineral density, as well as hip fracture and its sequelae[10]. HRT was assumed either to delay bone loss during the period of treatment (bone loss assumption) or to reduce the age-specific risk of hip fracture by 60% (epidemiologic assumption). Both risk-benefit and cost-effectiveness figures were calculated, the former from the perspective of individual patients, and the latter from the perspective of society at large. The analysis was based on a hypothetical population of women at menopause, averaging 50 years of age. Cardiovascular benefits of HRT were ignored in the model, and the same QoL assumptions as before were made, though they varied in the sensitivity analysis.

For a sequential combined HRT regime administered over a 15-year course, there is a net gain in QALE of 6.5 months with respect to no treatment, or over four months compared to a five-year combined treatment; the authors pointed out that symptom relief would add on top of that as a bonus. Dividing net lifetime costs by discounted future QALYs, translates into a CER ranging from $US 12 800–24 000

per gained QALY (with and without effect on QoL, respectively; 15 years of treatment compared with no treatment; 1988 US dollars) (Table 4). The authors concluded that HRT compares favorably to many widely accepted clinical practices, but point out that cost-effectiveness is highly dependent on (1) the treatment strategy considered; (2) the duration of treatment; and (3) the effect of treatment on QoL.

Daly and associates[11] introduced for the first time cardiovascular protection when assessing the cost-utility of ERT and HRT. Their analysis was constrained to a ten-year horizon and drug costs only include one conjugated equine estrogen (CEE) preparation. Costs were modeled with or without two-yearly endometrial biopsy. They highlighted that, in terms of net health benefits, the potential reduction in cardiovascular disease would have the greatest impact and would overshadow any small increase in breast cancer risk possibly associated with long-term use. For combined HRT in women with intact uteri, costs per QALY were £1900 for women with severe symptoms at baseline and £6200 for women with mild symptoms at baseline (in 1989/90 UK pounds sterling) and thus compare favorably with other accepted healthcare interventions. The same held true for long-term prophylactic ERT of hysterectomized women, be they symptomatic or not.

Cheung and Wren[12] amended Weinstein and Schiff's 1983 model[8] in that they optionally incorporated myocardial infarction (MI) as endpoint, alongside osteoporotic hip and wrist fracture. Gallbladder disease was

Table 6 Cost per QALY gained with different hormone replacement strategies in the indicated subgroups (1988 Australian dollars)

RR of death from MI	Symptomatic status	Women with intact uteri		Hysterectomized women
		E only	E + P	E only
1	symptoms	$15 100–17 500	$23 900–34 700 ($13 900–17 600)	$9530–12 300
	no symptoms	D*	$83 600–1 450 000	$57 100–1 020 000
0.75	symptoms	$11 800–14 900	$18 000–27 400 ($11 600–15 300)	$7800–10 700
	no symptoms	D*–205 500	$40 000–126 000	$27 200–87 900
0.5	symptoms	$9500–12 900	$14 300–22 400 ($9820–13 600)	$6510–9380
	no symptoms	$45 800–158 000	$26 100–64 800	$17 300–44 800

Lower and upper bounds represent 15 and 5 years of treatment, respectively; MI, myocardial infarction; RR, relative risk; E, estrogen; P, progestogen; figures in brackets assume no progestogen side-effects, i.e. no loss in QoL due to bleeding; *D, dominated strategy, i.e. 'no treatment' was preferable to treatment, as the latter would generate a net QALY loss and still incur costs

excluded from the model because newer studies showed its lack of association with HRT. Vertebral fracture was not considered in the analysis. QoL adjustments were the same as those used in the Weinstein and Schiff model (including the halved QoL gain when bleeding occurred), with the additional assumption of MI causing the same QoL loss as hip fracture (i.e. 0.05 QALY per remaining year of life). Regarding drug costs, and unlike previous groups, these researchers used the average price of several different oral formulations.

Cheung and Wren simulated a 5–15 year follow-up of all women aged 50 – the assumed age of natural menopause – in New South Wales, Australia ($n = 27 021$), comparing both HRT and ERT with 'no treatment' (see Table 6). After a careful discussion of the appropriateness of the utility assumptions, the cardiac benefits and the role of the progestogen in both of these, they suggested two sets of conclusions, one for symptomatic and one for asymptomatic women. For symptomatic women, and including a 50% risk reduction in mortality from MI, the authors argued that: (1) treatment with estrogen or estrogen and progestogen (assuming no progestogen side-effects) is an efficient use of healthcare resources – especially for a treatment duration of 15 years – yielding CER under $Aus 10 000/QALY; (2) in the presence of progestogen side-effects, long-term estrogen and progestogen treatment is still reasonably cost-effective (CER = $Aus 14 300/QALY); and (3) ERT after hysterectomy is cost-effective for all treatment durations, with CER ranging from $Aus 6510–9380 per QALY (Table 5). Conversely, including the same cardiac benefit but looking at asymptomatic women, the findings suggest that (1) long-term treatment with combined therapy (for women with intact uteri) is intermediate in CE; (2) prolonged ERT post-hysterectomy represents a reasonable use of resources; but that (3) short-term treatment is not particularly cost-effective.

Summarizing, they highlighted the factors associated with improved cost-effectiveness: prolonged treatment duration, the presence of menopausal symptoms, minimum progestogen side-effects in the case of combined regimens, estrogen-only use for women after hysterectomy, and inclusion of cardiac benefits (in addition to fracture prevention).

Until the mid-1990s, the most comprehensive CUA of HRT was the one by Tosteson and colleagues[13]. Their model included the expected annual impact of HRT on hip fractures and associated sequelae, nursing home admissions, heart disease mortality, breast cancer mortality and QoL. Though the model was rather complex, it still disregarded a number of cost components like the impact of indirect costs (such as foregone productivity), the reduction in healthcare costs resulting from decreased rates of heart disease in women receiving HRT, and the costs of any breast cancer treatment. The researchers' model estimated the costs and consequences of two populations: the first comprised 50-year-old women with intact uteri receiving CEE, 0.625 mg daily, plus MPA 5–10 mg on days 1–13 monthly for 10–15 years; and the second consisted of 50-year-old women with a previous hysterectomy receiving the same estrogen therapy (without the progestogen) for 10–15 years. The study used a Markov state-transition model and estimated the costs and consequences for women, who were initially well, from age 50 until their death or age 99. The key endpoints of the model are summarized in Box 2.

The net economic result of this hypothetical model indicated that the cost of HRT drugs and monitoring exceeded the cost savings resulting from fewer hip fractures and nursing home admissions. However, and as the authors point out, this was not unexpected: most

---

Net effectiveness (life expectancy)
  Coronary heart disease (CHD)-mortality
    decrease
  Osteoporotic hip fracture (OHF)-mortality
    decrease
  Possible breast cancer mortality increase

Quality of life adjustments
  Morbidity if hip fracture occurs
  Menopausal symptom relief
  Adverse effects from HRT

Net cost
  HRT costs (drugs and physician visits)
  Cost of long-term nursing home care saved
  Hip fracture treatment cost saved

Box 2 Cost, effectiveness and utility outcomes accounted for in the 1994 Tosteson and colleagues model[13] (reproduced with permission, Raven Press)

---

prophylactic therapies, such as the treatment of mild-to-moderate hypertension, would require a net increase in healthcare costs to achieve an improvement in clinical outcome. Accounting for savings generated from averted indirect costs and reduced cardiovascular morbidity in the economic model would reverse this finding; that is, if indirect and cardiovascular cost savings were included, long-term HRT might produce a net cost saving.

The cost-effectiveness results of the study estimated the cost per life-year (LY) saved to lie between $US 15 300–81 800. The cost per LY saved was lowest in women with a previous hysterectomy being treated for 15 years, and highest if an increased risk of breast cancer was assumed and patients were treated for only 10 years. In women treated with HRT for 15 years, if no increase in breast cancer was assumed, the cost per life-year saved was $US 23 900.

In the CUA – where LY were adjusted for QoL to yield QALYs – the CERs improved, reflecting reduced disability due to hip fractures and relief from menopausal symptoms. Table 7 lists the cost-per-QALY ratios for groups of women with various characteristics. This table demonstrates that women with menopausal symptoms who do not suffer from adverse HRT effects have the lowest CER; those who do have a slightly higher cost-per-QALY ratio.

The reader should be aware that evidence on the degree to which menopausal symptoms alter the different domains or dimensions of QoL remains inconclusive, even today. All of the afore-mentioned studies rely on hypothetical QoL weights assigned to different health states and are, as Zethraeus and colleagues[5] put it, "qualified guesses rather than based on empirical data". Rigorous empirical research in this area is highly desirable given that cost-per-QALY ratios are highly sensitive to the utility adjustments used.

Recognition of the need for empirical QoL assessment

In 1993, Daly and co-workers[14] were the first to actually measure the impact of menopausal

Table 7 Cost per QALY (in 1992 US dollars) according to the 1994 Tosteson and colleagues model[13] (reproduced with permission, Raven Press)

Patient group	HRT adverse effects	Model assumption	
		No breast cancer risk with HRT	Breast cancer risk with HRT
Symptomatic	yes	$11 600	$16 600
	no	$9700	$13 000
Non-symptomatic	yes	$26 300	$70 000
	no	$17 900	$32 000

Women with intact uterus on combined HRT, 15-year treatment course, level of symptoms or frequency of endometrial biopsies not stated

symptoms on QoL on a utility basis, using the time trade-off (TTO) technique and a rating scale (visual analogue scale, VAS) approach. The former is a preference-based measure and places the respondent in an explicit decision-making context. Supported by graphical illustration, each woman is asked to choose between living with her current health for her remaining statistical life expectancy (x) or living for fewer years (y) in perfect health. The number of these fewer years is varied until reaching the point of indifference between the two options, the resulting ratio y/x representing the utility value attached to her current health state. For example, if a woman's life expectancy was 20 years and she were indifferent between living those 20 years in her current health and living for only 15 years (i.e. giving up five years of life) in perfect health, the remaining 20 years of LE would be equivalent to 15 QALYs; the utility value attached to her current health status is 15/20 = 0.75.

A VAS is a simple vertical numerical scale from 0–10 with defined end points of death and full health. Both techniques – TTO and VAS – used the same descriptions of menopausal symptoms, which were split in two sets, one describing mild and another describing severe symptoms. These included hot flushes, night sweats, concentration, self-confidence, tiredness and dyspareunia.

Though poorly related, both measures were consistent – producing much lower utility scores than those assumed in the previous models, specifically 0.85 and 0.65 for mild symptoms, and 0.64 and 0.3 for severe menopausal symptoms (TTO and VAS-generated scores, respectively). Given the preference-based – and hence, more 'purist' – nature of the TTO method, the TTO values can generally be given greater faith[15]. Box 3 shows further assumptions of the model.

Zethraeus and co-workers[5] carried out a similar study on 104 Swedish women aged 45–65 years. In order to assess the QoL impact of menopausal symptoms and HRT, they used the VAS, TTO and WTP approaches. Both the VAS and the TTO-generated QoL gains are very much in line with the results of the Daly group[14]: TTO-derived scores indicate a QoL gain of 0.18 utils for women with mild symptoms and of 0.42 utils for those with severe symptoms.

Neither study can exclude the problems of selection and recall bias; that is, neither can address how representative the participating women were of the general menopausal population, or to what extent women's recollection of their state before HRT was accurate.

Tosteson and associates[16] empirically derived QALY gains for current HRT users relative to never- and past users. In this study only the QoL impact of fracture prevention and of HRT-borne side-effects were modeled. The positive influence of HRT on menopausal symptoms was not evaluated. Using a TTO-based automated instrument, they derived an overall gain in QALYs ranging from 15–83.7 days per year of treatment in HRT users, with

QoL gain due to HRT
- Women with mild symptoms   plus (1–0.85) = 0.15 utils (or 0.15 QALYs per year of HRT)
- Women with severe symptoms   plus (1–0.64) = 0.36 utils (or 0.36 QALYs per year of HRT)

Duration of symptoms, i.e. time for which HRT users would experience symptom relief   Four years, regardless of severity of symptoms

Proportion of symptomatic women who experience
- symptom relief   90%
- no change in QoL   5%
- side-effects   5%

QoL reduction due to side-effects   Minus 0.3 QALY per year of treatment

HRT continuation in case of side-effects   Six months

Box 3 Key assumptions in the assessment of the impact of menopausal symptoms and HRT on quality of life. Mild and severe symptoms were empirically shown to correspond to utility levels of 0.85 and 0.64, respectively.

respect to never- or past users. Over a 15-year period of HRT, these would generate 225–1255.5 days of extra QALE, i.e. between 0.6 and 3.4 QALYs – on average, about four times higher than derived by Weinstein and Tosteson[9] ten years earlier. Benefits were largest for women with a vertebral fracture and limitations in their activities. Undesirable effects of HRT can be rank-ordered as bleeding, breast tenderness, weight gain and endometrial biopsy, their importance being reflected by the number of days of life women were prepared to forego in order to avoid them.

The empirical evidence – despite its obvious shortcomings – suggests that the burden of menopausal symptoms on QoL may have been underestimated in pharmaco-economic analyses in the past[5,17]. Consequently, previous economic studies may have underestimated the value of HRT[16].

Modern health economic models

Based on their empirically derived QoL weights, Daly and colleagues[18] performed a CUA of estrogen-only and combined estrogen–progestogen therapy, given to hysterectomized and non-hysterectomized women, respectively. The base case assumed treatment for ten years,

with full compliance, starting at age 50. Two extra annual GP visits were assumed for users. A breakdown of collected variables is given in Box 4.

Based on the assumptions in the model, the analysis produced the results for the treatment of mildly symptomatic women as shown in Table 8.

The authors emphasize that there is "a dramatic reduction in cost per life year gained when adjustments are made for symptom relief". For combined therapy users (ten-year treatment), the cost falls from £17 700 per non-QALY to less than £1000 when adjustments are made for QoL improvements.

The same TTO-based QoL weights (0.85 and 0.64 for mild and severe symptoms, respectively) are used in a recent study assessing the cost-utility of tibolone[19]. In this analysis, tibolone is compared to 'no treatment' and to continuous combined HRT (ccHRT). Only symptom alleviation is considered as a source of QoL gains; preventive effects are not considered, and side-effects are only indirectly accounted for as they differentially influence continuation rates. The author assumed the same potential QoL gains (+ 0.15 or + 0.36 utils for alleviating mild and severe symptoms, respectively) to be reaped from either tibolone or ccHRT. The

5

Overall consequences of therapy
- Mortality induced or prevented by HRT
- Morbidity induced or prevented by HRT
- Changes in QoL following relief of menopausal symptoms
- Healthcare costs associated with treatment

Disease endpoints considered (ICD9 code)
- Endometrial cancer (179, 182)
- Breast cancer (174)
- Fractured neck of femur (820, 821)
- Fractured wrist (814)
- Fractured vertebra (805)
- Ischemic heart disease (410–414)
- Stroke (430–438)

Healthcare cost components
- Expected lifetime cost of therapy (including monitoring and maintenance costs)
- Expected costs of treating side-effects
- Expected savings from reduced morbidity
- Expected costs of treating patients during any increased life expectancy

---

Box 4 Costs and effects associated to HRT use considered in the 1996 Daly *et al.* model[18] (reproduced with permission, *Maturitas*

Table 8 Cost per QALY for different periods with estrogen only or estrogen plus progestogen, assuming five years of relief from mild menopausal symptoms. (Costs in 1992 UK pounds sterling)

	Estrogen-only	Estrogen plus progestogen
5-year treatment period	£310	£550
10-year treatment period	£490	£900
15-year treatment period	£600	£1110
20-year treatment period	£660	£1250

differentiation lies in the probabilities used to model costs and consequences through the underlying decision–analytic framework. Tibolone is assumed to have lower discontinuation rates than ccHRT – see Table 9 for reasons of discontinuation and their corresponding probablities.

Integrating continuation rates and potential QoL gains, so-called 'expected' QoL gains were computed, and were higher for the tibolone group. The author modeled the cost-utility over the time horizons of one and five years, using one-year discontinuation rates in four alternative scenarios (one for each reason of discontinuation) of the five-year time horizon. Table 10 summarizes the cost and QALY values for a one-year, overall discontinuation scenario. The resulting CERs are given in Table 11. Tibolone's incremental cost-effectiveness ratios with respect to ccHRT are considerably higher than its CERs compared to no intervention, which can be interpreted as the markup price to pay for an extra unit of effect. The author concludes, however, that tibolone compares favorably to ccHRT on health economic grounds.

Armstrong and colleagues[21] recently modelled a further drug-to-drug comparison. They used a sample of 30 Philadelphia-based internists to assign utility weights to various

Table 9 Likelihood of one-year discontinuation with tibolone and continuous combined HRT due to various reasons. Data originally from Hammar *et al.*, 1998[20] (reproduced with permission, *British Journal of Obstetrics and Gynaecology*)

	Tibolone	*ccHRT*
Overall	0.25	0.31
Side-effects	0.16	0.25
Bleeding and breast tenderness	0.02	0.16
Bleeding	0.02	0.13

Table 10 QALY gains and drug costs. Overall discontinuation rate, one year time horizon (reproduced with permission, *British Journal of Obstetrics and Gynaecology*)

	Tibolone vs. no treatment	*Combined HRT vs. no treatment*	*Tibolone vs. combined HRT*
QALY gains			
Mild symptoms	0.113	0.103	0.01
Severe symptoms	0.270	0.248	0.022
Drug cost (1998 UK pounds)	£164	£104 (E + NETA) £91 (CE+MPA)	£60 £73

Table 11 Cost (in 1998 UK pounds) per QALY of tibolone compared with no treatment and continuous combined HRT under the overall discontinuation rate assumption and a one-year treatment period

	Tibolone vs no treatment	*Tibolone vs ccHRT*
Mild symptoms	164/0.113 = £1450	60/0.01 = £6000 73/0.01 = £7300
Severe symptoms	164/0.270 = £607	60/0.022 = £2730 73/0.022 = £3320

Comparison of tibolone to ccHRT yields a so-called incremental CER (ICER), as the extra cost per extra QALYs is being calculated

health states (Table 12). The Markov-model-based analysis compared the following regimens: HRT (0.625 mg of oral CE per day with cyclic progestin); raloxifene (60 mg per day); and no therapy. The simulation included both quality-adjusted and unadjusted LE. Only direct medical costs were included. The base case assumed women to be 50 years of age at baseline, have an average risk of heart disease and breast cancer, to be fully compliant and to take lifetime therapy; future costs and outcomes were discounted at 3%. These assumptions were subsequently altered in the sensitivity analysis. The results of the base case are shown in Table 13.

It can bee seen that – for a woman at average risk of breast cancer and CHD – lifetime HRT yields greater gains in QALE (1.75 compared with 1.32 QALYs) and costs less than raloxifene (US\$ 3802 compared with 12 968), thus making it the 'dominant' strategy. The sensitivity analysis, where relative risks and treatment duration were varied, could show that raloxifene is more cost-effective for women with a lifetime breast cancer risk of 15% or higher, or who receive only ten years or less of therapy. Raloxifene would also be more cost-effective if CHD protection from HRT is less than 20%. The authors therefore conclude that, assuming the CHD prevention benefit of HRT shown in observational studies, HRT is the most cost-effective alternative for women at average breast cancer and CHD risk who wish to extend their QALE after menopause. However, raloxifene was the more cost-effective alternative for women at average CHD risk but one or more major breast cancer risk factors (first-degree relative, prior breast biopsy, atypical hyperplasia or BRCA1/2 mutation).

The most comprehensive and flexible model published to date appears to be the one by Zethraeus and colleagues[22,23]. The authors thoroughly described a Markov model based on ten health states, outlining its structure and data requirements. Each health state is characterized by age-specific costs, mortality rates and QoL weights. The relative risks used are either tabulated figures or are imputed by risk functions. The increased risk of breast

Table 12 Utility estimates assigned to health conditions (in different years) by 30 Philadelphia internists[21] (reproduced with permission, *Obstetrics and Gynaecology*)

Condition	Utility estimate
CHD	
First year	0.665
Subsequent years	0.871
Death year	0.274
Breast cancer	
First year	0.546
Subsequent years	0.864
Death year	0.192
Hip fracture	
First year	0.613
Subsequent years	0.915
Vertebral fracture	
First year	0.704
Subsequent years	0.858
Endometrial cancer	
First year	0.577
Subsequent years	0.881
Death year	0.192
Thromboembolism	
First year	0.682
Subsequent years	0.925

Table 13 Results of the base case analysis by Armstrong and colleagues[21] (reproduced with permission, *Obstetrics and Gynaecology*)

Time frame	Strategy*	Δ LYs	Δ QALYs	Δ cost (US$)	Incremental CER (Δ $/Δ QALYs)
Long-term therapy	**HRT** vs. No therapy	0.65	1.75	3802	2173
	Raloxifene vs. no therapy	0.71	1.32	12 968	9824
	Raloxifene vs. HRT	0.06	−0.43	9166	HRT dominant**
Ten-year therapy	**HRT** vs. no therapy	0.36	0.90	3834	4260
	Raloxifene vs. no therapy	0.47	1.03	8123	7886
	Raloxifene vs. HRT	0.11	0.13	4289	32 992
Five-year therapy	**HRT** vs. no therapy	0.16	0.45	2259	5020
	Raloxifene vs. no therapy	0.28	0.52	851	9328
	Raloxifene vs. HRT	0.12	0.07	2592	37 029

*Strategy in bold represents the most cost-effective alternative; **more effective while less costly

cancer used was 0 or 35%, with the risk increase assumed to start instantaneously after five years of treatment (five years start delay, zero rise time) and remain elevated (only) during the rest of treatment. All data inputs, except the majority of QoL weights, stem from empirical investigation. The origin or values of utility weights used in the QALY calculations are not explicitly stated, but are reported to take into account both morbidity and side-effects.

Characteristically, the revised version of the model relies entirely on Swedish data, which circumvents the question of data transferability between countries; however, in the conclusions, the authors point out that the use of Framingham data for CHD risk in the original model was warranted and produced similar results. The basic model assumes an initially healthy cohort (the size of which can vary between 1 and 100 000) of age 50, 60 or 70. Costs and consequences of a ten-year treatment course are modeled over the remaining life expectancy (operational-ized by age 110 in the model).

A particular strength of the model is that it adopts a full societal perspective, i.e. all costs are measured, no matter who bears them. These include direct costs, indirect costs and costs in added life years. Direct costs are those directly related to treatment (drug costs, physician visits, hospital services), indirect costs represent productivity losses (due to work absenteeism) and costs in added life years are equal to total consumption minus total production in those years. From an operational point of view, the cost inputs into the model are divided into intervention, morbidity and mortality costs. Intervention costs include the cost of the HRT preparation and physician visits (yearly costs) as well as the cost of pre-treatment screening. Morbidity costs represent the aggregate of costs incurred due to increased morbidity from breast cancer minus costs saved because of reduced morbidity (from CHD and fractures). Mortality costs, in turn, represent the net of total consumption minus total production due to a change in mortality attributed to the intervention. The estimation of total consumption and produc-

tion is typically based on a healthy population, free from fractures, breast cancer and CHD.

Table 14 gives an overview of the CERs for different risk assumptions and different ages of treatment onset. Assuming a 20% reduction in risk of CHD, CER improves with age at treatment onset. The improved CERs are mainly explained by an increased absolute risk of CHD as age increases and, therefore, a larger decrease in the number of CHD events and related mortality compared with HRT at younger ages. There is also an age-related absolute risk of breast cancer and fractures, but not as large as for CHD.

Assuming a 50% reduction in the risk of CHD, the CER increases with age in some cases. With low CERs at the age of 50 years, an increase in the effectiveness of starting treatment in older ages result in higher CERs, due to costs in added life-years; the costs incurred during added life-years are large above 65 years of age, for which the increase in costs outweighs the increase in LE for the ratio calculation. By adding the risk of breast cancer, the CER generally worsens. This is due to a lower LE and decreased savings in morbidity costs. However, due to the lower LE, costs in added LYs also diminish, which in turn leads to a decrease in total cost, and hence a slight decrease of the CER is observed in some cases.

This analysis, too, shows that CERs are sensitive to (1) the magnitude of risk reduction from CHD; (2) the risk of breast cancer; and (3) any QoL adjustments (in either sense). Allowing for side-effects, HRT may be dominated by the 'no treatment' alternative in some cases. However, and by the same token, CER also improves substantially when adjusting for the relief of menopausal symptoms. Adding the assumption that spine and wrist fracture exactly follow the risk profile of hip fracture only slightly changed CERs in this model.

CONCLUSIONS AND OUTLOOK

This review has given an impression of how health economic analyses of HRT developed over time, with special attention to both their potential and their limitations. Study limita-

Table 14 Cost (SEK thousand) per LY gained (per QALY gained, in parenthesis) assuming different risk reductions for CHD, fracture, and breast cancer. The treatment duration is ten years, administered to women aged 50, 60 and 70 years. Analysis based on the revised version of the computer model[23] (reproduced with permission)

Risk change	E only (post-hysterectomy)			E+P (intact uterus)		
	50	60	70	50	60	70
Fra −40%	8460 (1350)	950 (430)	210 (170)	12 230 (1960)	1470 (670)	330 (270)
Fra −40%, CHD −20%	480 (370)	240 (230)	170 (190)	700 (540)	320 (300)	200 (230)
Fra −40%, CHD −50%	200 (180)	180 (190)	160 (200)	290 (260)	210 (220)	170 (220)
Fra −50%	6330 (1010)	660 (300)	140 (110)	9350 (1500)	1080 (490)	240 (190)
Fra −50%, CHD −20%	440 (330)	220 (200)	150 (170)	660 (480)	290 (270)	180 (200)
Fra −50%, CHD −50%	190 (160)	170 (170)	150 (180)	270 (240)	200 (210)	160 (200)
Fra −40%, cancer +35%	D (D)	D (1270)	260 (140)	D (D)	D (2380)	500 (280)
Fra −40%, CHD −20%, cancer +35%	D (1110)	290 (240)	170 (190)	D (1830)	400 (330)	210 (230)
Fra −40%, CHD −50%, cancer +35%	280 (200)	180 (190)	160 (200)	470 (320)	220 (220)	180 (220)
Fra −50%, cancer +35%	D (D)	D (460)	130 (80)	D (D)	D (970)	290 (180)
Fra −50%, CHD −20%, cancer +35%	D (780)	250 (200)	150 (160)	D (1330)	350 (280)	180 (200)
Fra −50%, CHD −50%, cancer +35%	250 (170)	170 (170)	150 (180)	440 (290)	200 (210)	170 (200)

E, estrogen; P, progestogen; Fra, fracture (hip, spine, wrist); CHD, coronary heart disease; cancer, breast cancer; D, dominated strategy – here, 'no treatment' is the better alternative as treating would confer net loss in LYs/QALYs (and still cost money); SEK, Swedish kronor (SEK 1000 = US$90.56 or £64.77 on 07 July

tions are not unique to the field of health economic evaluation, and are most often attributable to the lack of suitable data. Comprehensive, reality-mimicking models are desirable, although increasing complexity may complicate the interpretation of results for a non-expert audience.

Health economic models are particularly data-hungry, such that assumptions are an unavoidable fact of life. Sensitivity analysis can address the issues of uncertainty surrounding critical data assumptions. The ideal pharmaco-economic appraisal of HRT in menopausal women would assess the influence of all risks and benefits; consider the effectiveness of different treatment regimens for all types and degrees of menopausal symptoms, urogenital deficiency and osteoporotic fracture; evaluate the effect of different compliance levels over treatment durations; and adjust the outcomes with respect to QoL. Indirect costs could optionally be included according to prevailing population characteristics (employment, wage rate), and different sets of discount rates for costs and benefits could be applied. With little agreement in the literature concerning the optimum duration of treatment, levels of compliance and QoL effects of HRT, the ideal appraisal is still elusive at present[24].

The lack of randomized controlled studies on natural endpoints – for example fractures rather than bone mineral density and markers of bone turnover; cardiovascular disease and stroke rather than blood lipids – further compounds this problem. As a matter of fact, HRT-mediated cardiovascular protection has come under crossfire in the light of the results from the Heart and Estrogen/progestin Replacement Study (HERS) trial[25]. If HRT were ultimately found not to be cardioprotective, its cost-effectiveness would decrease considerably. But the current evidence is inconclusive. First and foremost, with HERS being a secondary prevention trial, its results cannot be applied to the use of HRT in the primary prevention of CHD. The HERS cohort had a mean age of 67 years at treatment onset and did not exclude other co-morbid conditions. Secondly, the findings cannot be expected to apply to the full range of natural or synthetic hormones, strengths and regimens.

Nevertheless, the review of pharmaco-economic assessments has highlighted the factors that are of particular importance to an enhanced cost-effectiveness and cost-utility of HRT: patient characteristics, treatment attributes and model assumptions. Regarding patient characteristics, hormone treatment should be prescribed – on cost-effectiveness or cost-utility grounds – to those women who suffer from mild or severe symptoms, have undergone hysterectomy and are at high or intermediate risk of fractures and/or CHD. Minimum progestogen side-effects, long-term treatment continuation (ten years or more) and high compliance rates further improve CERs.

In terms of model assumptions, the factors that will considerably affect CERs are the perspective, the time horizon considered and the QoL weights used, apart from the obviously important risk assumptions. Concerning the perspective, a full societal perspective (including all costs and benefits associated to therapy, no matter to whom they accrue) should be adopted, rather then a healthcare payer perspective. As far as the time horizon is concerned, preference should be given to lifetime costs and consequences (no matter whether or not HRT is being given during all that time) rather then pre-set, say, ten-year time frames. Finally, more research is needed into the integrated QoL impact of menopausal symptoms, adverse affects of HRT, and its long-term complications if they occur. Preference-based measures are particularly suitable for this as they allow women to trade-off all individually perceived effects against each other. Research into this field is currently being undertaken by Zöllner and associates[26].

It should be said that real-life decisions regarding the implementation of an intervention for a given population are rarely based solely on economic grounds. Ethical and political motivations are also to be considered. While the economic rationale is to maximize total health gains subject to a given budget constraint, politics is about maximizing voter support for certain healthcare decisions; equity, in turn, is concerned with maximizing fairness in access to healthcare interventions.

As far as cost-effectiveness and cost-utility are concerned, professional deontology of researchers, clinicians and payers alike mandate the objective use and pursuit of up-to-date health economic evidence in the best interest of patients and the healthcare system as a whole. Future challenges for the conduct and acceptance of health economic studies of HRT will include the undertaking of long-term studies with natural endpoints, the empirical derivation of quality-of-life data, and the appropriate use of modeling.

References

1. Kavanos P, Trueman P, Bosilevac A. Can economic evaluation guidelines improve efficiency in resource allocation? The cases of Portugal, The Netherlands, Finland and the UK. *LSE Health, London School of Economics and Political Science, discussion paper 15*, January 2000
2. Jacobzone S. *Pharmaceutical Policies in OECD Countries: Reconciling. Social and Industrial goals. Labor Market and Social Policy – Occasional Papers*, number 40. Paris: OECD Publications Service, 2000
3. Lerner BH. Body politics – how public pressure, private interests and powerful lobbies infect the treatment of breast cancer. *The Washington Post* (Suppl) May 22, 2001:1–5
4. Graf von der Schulenburg JM, Hoffmann C. Review of European guidelines for economic evaluation of medical technologies and pharmaceuticals. *Health Economics in Prevention and Care (HEPAC)* 2000;1:2–8
5. Zethraeus N, Johannesson M, Henriksson P, *et al.* The impact of hormone replacement therapy on quality of life and willingness to pay. *Br J Obstet Gynaecol* 1997;104:1191–5
6. Francis RM, Anderson FH, Torgerson DJ. A comparison of the effectiveness and cost of treatment for vertebral fractures in women. *Br J Rheumatol* 1995;34:1167–71
7. Weinstein M. Estrogen use in postmenopausal women – costs, risks and benefits. *N Engl J Med* 1980;303:308–16
8. Weinstein MC, Schiff I. Cost-effectiveness of hormone replacement therapy in the menopause. *Obstet Gynecol Surv* 1983;38:445–55
9. Weinstein MC, Tosteson ANA. Cost-effectiveness of hormone replacement. *Ann N Y Acad Sci* 1990;593:162–72
10. Melton LJ, Wahner HW, Richelson LS, *et al.* Osteoporosis and the risk of hip fracture. *Am J Epidemiol* 1986;124:254–61
11. Daly E, Roche M, Barlow D, *et al.* HRT: an analysis of benefits, risks and costs. *Br Med Bull* 1992;48:368–400
12. Cheung AP, Wren BG. A cost-effectiveness analysis of hormone replacement therapy in the menopause. *Med J Aust* 1992;156:312–16
13. Tosteson AN, Weinstein MC, Schiff I. Cost-effectiveness analysis of hormone replacement therapy. In: Lobo RA, ed. *Treatment of the Postmenopausal Woman: Basic and Clinical Aspects.* New York: Raven Press, 1994:405–13
14. Daly E, Gray A, Barlow D, *et al.* Measuring the impact of menopausal symptoms on quality of life. *Br Med J* 1993;307:836–40
15. Dolan P. Valuing health-related quality of life.
16. Tosteson ANA, Gabriel S, Kneeland T, *et al.* Has the impact of hormone replacement therapy on health-related quality of life been undervalued? *J Womens Health Gend Based Med* 2000; 9:119–30
17. Whittington R, Faulds D. Hormone replacement therapy: I. A pharmacoeconomic appraisal of its therapeutic use in menopausal symptoms and urogenital estrogen deficiency. *Pharmacoeconomics* 1994;5:419–45
18. Daly E, Vessey MP, Barlow D, *et al.* Hormone replacement therapy in a risk-benefit perspective. *Maturitas* 1996;23:247–59
19. Phillips CJ. Livial: an economic appraisal. *Br J Obstet Gynaecol* 1999;106(S19):22–8
20. Hammar M, Christau S, Nathorst-Boos J, *et al.* A double-blind, randomised trial comparing the effects of tibolone and continuous hormone replacement therapy in postmenopausal women with menopausal symptoms. *Br J Obstet Gynaecol* 1998;105:904–11
21. Armstrong K, Chen TM, Albert D, *et al.* Cost-effectiveness of raloxifene and hormone replacement therapy in postmenopausal women: impact of breast cancer risk. *Obstet Gynecol* 2001; 6:996–1003
22. Zethraeus N, Johannesson M, Jonsson B. A computer model to analyse the cost-effectiveness of hormone replacement therapy. *Int J Technol Assess Health Care* 1999;15:352–65
23. Zethraeus N, Lindgren P, Johnell O, *et al.* A computer model to analyse the cost-effectiveness of hormone replacement therapy – a revised version. *Stockholm School of Economics, SSE/EFI Working Paper series in Economics and Finance, No 368*, March 2000
24. Whittington R, Faulds D. Hormone replacement therapy: II. A pharmacoeconomic appraisal of its role in the prevention of postmenopausal osteoporosis and ischaemic heart disease. *Pharmacoeconomics* 1994;5:513–54
25. Hulley S, Grady D, Bush T, *et al.* Randomized trial of estrogen plus progestin for secondary prevention of coronary heart disease in postmenopausal women. Heart and Estrogen/progestin Replacement Study (HERS) Research Group. *J Am Med Assoc* 1998;280:605–13
26. Zöllner YF, Brazier JE, Oliver P, *et al.* Development of an algorithm to derive utilities from a validated menopause-specific QoL questionnaire (paper discussion). 59th Health Economists' Study Group (HESG) meeting, London, 2001

Issues and controversies. *Pharmacoeconomics* 1998;15:119–27

Index